A Noted Pediatrician's Most Valuable Advice...

"The best time to learn about the new baby is before it is born. Having all your questions answered ahead of time will make things that much easier. It will allow you to relax and enjoy your new baby when it arrives.

"The HANDBOOK FOR NEW PARENTS is my way of educating mothers and fathers...

"You will know when to stop worrying about the wrong things so that you can relax and enjoy your baby. That is what good parenting is all about. And that is the kind of parent you will become after reading this book."

* * *

Dr. Alvin N. Eden, M.D., is Director of Pediatrics at a Brooklyn, NY, hospital, and author of the bestselling *Growing Up Thin*. In addition, he maintains an active private pediatric practice.

HANDBOOK FOR NEW PARENTS

ALVIN N. EDEN, M.D.

A BERKLEY BOOK
published by
BERKLEY PUBLISHING CORPORATION

Much of the material in the *Handbook for New Parents* first appeared in *American Baby* magazine.

HANDBOOK FOR NEW PARENTS

A Berkley Book/published by arrangement with
the author

PRINTING HISTORY
Berkley Medallion edition published January 1978
Berkley edition/November 1979

All rights reserved.
Copyright © 1978 by Alvin N. Eden, M.D.
Foreword Copyright © 1978 by Vincent J. Montana, M.D.
This book may not be reproduced in whole or in part, by mimeograph or any other means, without permission. For information address:

Berkley Publishing Corporation
200 Madison Avenue
New York, New York 10016

ISBN: 0-425-04285-5

A BERKLEY BOOK ® TM 757,375

PRINTED IN THE UNITED STATES OF AMERICA

DEDICATION

For my wife Elaine

and

our children, Robert and Elizabeth

—with all my love

ACKNOWLEDGMENTS

For their comments and ideas I would like to thank my editors at Berkley, Page Cuddy and Betsy Nordstrom.

For her support and cooperation I am grateful to Judith Nolte, the Editor of *American Baby* magazine.

I especially want to thank my secretary, Catherine Hayes, for her untiring efforts and continuous calm optimism.

AUTHOR'S NOTE

As I stated in my previous book, *Growing Up Thin*, I firmly believe in the equality of the sexes. Because the English language provides no graceful words to substitute for "his" and "her," or "he" and "she," I have decided to alternate the pronouns used to describe gender chapter by chapter, giving equal time to both sexes. Please remember, however, that these pronouns refer to your child, even if your baby is of the opposite sex—except, of course, where I make remarks that apply specifically to boys or girls. I start off in the first chapter with the pronoun "she," a decision made by the flip of a coin.

CONTENTS

Foreword by Vincent J. Montana, M.D.	1
Introduction	5
You and Your Baby's Doctor	9
How to Pick Your Baby's Doctor	11
Why the Monthly Visit?	18
When to Call Your Doctor	23
Immunizations	29
What to Expect as Your Baby Grows and Develops	35
The First Month	37
Feeding	43
Sleep	53
Crying	59
Pacifiers	64
Thumb Sucking	70
Teething	76
Accident Prevention	82
Toilet Training	90
The Role of the New Father	96
Should a Mother Go Back to Work?	101
Common Problems and What to Do about Them	107
Diaper Rash	109
Colic	114
Vomiting	118

Constipation	124
Diarrhea	129
Temperature	137
Fever	142
Fever Convulsions	147
The Common Cold	153
Breath Holding	159
Head Injuries	163
Jaundice in the Newborn	167
Answers to Questions Mothers Most Frequently Ask	173
Questions and Answers	175
Epilogue	205
Index	207

HANDBOOK FOR NEW PARENTS

FOREWORD

Vincent J. Fontana, M.D.

Medical Director and Pediatrician-in-Chief, New York Foundling Hospital Center for Parent and Child Development; Professor of Clinical Pediatrics, New York University College of Medicine; Author of *SOMEWHERE A CHILD IS CRYING*. Mentor Books, New York, 1976.

The HANDBOOK FOR NEW PARENTS, based on Dr. Eden's many years of experience as a practicing pediatrician and a practicing parent, is a remarkable achievement. By answering all the questions a parent could conceivably ask about the new baby, Dr. Eden has succeeded in taking the worry out of caring for an infant. The HANDBOOK FOR NEW PARENTS answers those questions parents worry about most and can't find discussed in other works. It is a unique book in that it can be read by those who are thinking about having a baby, as well as parents with newborn infants and mothers and fathers whose child is beginning the learning years. It is truly an essential book for all parents—one that will make the parenting experience more deeply satisfying and personally enriching.

Parenting, as Dr. Eden knows, is not a natural state. We are not born with the knowledge of how to be good parents, and frequently we are not even given the opportunity to learn or to observe how to be good parents from relatives, family or friends. Frequently, we do not live in the kind of tight-knit community where mothers, grandmothers or grandfathers teach their sons and daughters what crying means, when it is time to start a baby on solid foods, or how to know when a baby is well. These are the kinds of questions that are not magically answered at the same time a child is born, and that's why Dr. Eden's book is so valuable.

All of us wish to give our children the best. And the best you can give any child is not material possessions but spiritual and emotional strength. This kind of support begins with knowing how to care for your child in a physical sense. The knowledge of how to raise your child confidently allows you the freedom to relax and simply give your baby the love he or she needs.

For normal growth and development a child must feel wanted, must be loved, and must be guided and encouraged to learn right from wrong. One can easily see why parenting is such an important, full-time, sometimes difficult, job. On the other hand, it can be a most rewarding experience. Dr. Eden provides just such help in learning how to fulfill a child's needs—emotional, social, intellectual and physical.

Frequently today, parents, mothers and fathers, are on their own. The everyday responsibilities of parenting may become frustrating, leading to anxiety and a feeling of loneliness—of being afraid to admit to ourselves and to others that we are having problems in child-rearing. The basic components of good parenting must include both verbal and nonverbal communication with your child, stimulation, and provision for adequate affection, love and nurturing.

All parents as well as all children are unique and different. Their human needs must be and can be mutually satisfied. The HANDBOOK FOR NEW PARENTS takes both the parent and the child into consideration, showing you how to stop worrying about your child and thus allowing you the freedom to fulfill your own life.

I congratulate Dr. Eden on this outstanding accomplishment, filling a long-neglected need for clear, concise, easy-to-read information on how to care for your baby. It is a unique book and one that no parent or prospective parent should be without.

INTRODUCTION

The *Handbook for New Parents* is based on my more than twenty years of experience as a practicing pediatrician. I enjoy my work today just as much as I did when I treated my first baby at University Hospital in New York City over twenty years ago. In spite of the long, sometimes exhausting, hours involved, all the crying and screaming I hear, and the endless time I spend answering telephone calls, I am happy that I chose to become a pediatrician. For me, there is nothing more fulfilling than helping people raise happy, healthy children. I believe that there is nothing more important in this world than our children. Good parenting is thus the most important job you will ever have.

I want my patients to be able to enjoy being parents. If they do, I am convinced that their children will have a big head start toward a happy, healthy, and self-sufficient future. I take pride and pleasure in the job of bringing up their babies in the best way possible.

In recent years, however, I have become more and

more troubled by the confusion, guilt, and tension so many parents live with as they go about the job of raising their infants. I am convinced that much of this unhappiness is simply due to a lack of basic knowledge about what to expect. The best time to learn about the new baby is before it is born. Having all your questions answered ahead of time will make things that much easier. It will allow you to relax and enjoy your new baby when it arrives. New parents certainly do try their very best, and although they may be intelligent and eager to give their baby the best of care, they are often misinformed or just plain uninformed. This lack of information leads to all sorts of misconceptions and problems.

The *Handbook for New Parents* is my solution. It answers just about all the important questions that I have been asked over and over again through the years.

Every baby needs a relaxed, happy environment in which to grow and develop. But sad to say, I just don't see this kind of atmosphere being created often enough. Rather, too many of the new mothers and fathers I deal with are irritable, tired, and chock-full of guilt. Instead of being able to really enjoy and have fun with the marvelous new member of the family, they fret about all sorts of unimportant matters. They just don't know what is normal for their baby, and they use up all sorts of energy in the wrong directions.

There is no reason to be frightened about bringing up a baby. A newborn baby is a sturdy and vigorous little being. Each one is a little different. Each varies within normal ranges and has individual, uniquely lovable characteristics. But parents must be informed and knowledgeable about what to expect about their infant's behavior patterns and bodily functions. Getting off to a good start will pay tremendous dividends later on. A relaxed, calm household is what all of us thrive on, our new babies included.

A fast look at the Contents will give you an idea of the kind of knowledge I am talking about. The subjects I discuss and the questions I answer are not about specific disease entities. New parents worry about things like colic, feedings, sleep, crying, etc. Too often they worry needlessly about these subjects simply because they do not know enough about them. Take my word for it, you really are not a failure as a parent if your baby has a diaper rash or is constipated. All children experience these problems, and it is not a sign that you have done something wrong if they do.

The first few months of a baby's life are extremely important for its healthy emotional development. Patterns of behavior are established very early. A healthy, relaxed start for both the baby and his parents is the single most important gift you can give your child. No one denies that there is a lot of hard work involved in raising a new baby, but you must never lose sight of the fact that your baby requires love and affection right from the start. If you are always agitated and worried, it is difficult to convey a relaxed, happy attitude to your child. By allaying much of the unnecessary anxiety caused by ignorance, you will be amazed by the extra time and energy you will have left over to love and enjoy your baby. And, if you start off on the right foot, chances are that you will be better able to help your child grow and develop into the happy, self-reliant person you hope to nurture.

The *Handbook for New Parents* is a book written for the 1970s. Now more than ever, prospective parents and new parents need direction and help in raising their infants and giving them quality care. Our difficult contemporary times put a great deal of extra pressure on the family structure. Divorce, single parenthood, and child abuse are all around us. I am convinced that learning to appreciate and enjoy the enchanting newest member of your family right from the start is one of the keys to strengthening and solidifying the family unit.

There is no job more important than raising a happy, healthy baby, and it takes more than just common sense to do so. You also need to learn to separate the facts from the fiction. Our school systems unfortunately do not include courses in parenting. I hope that this book will help to bridge the gap in our education. I have attempted to lay to rest once and for all many myths and old wives' tales, and I have done my best to present the material simply so that it can be easily understood by everybody. It is arranged so that you can turn right to the information you need.

The *Handbook for New Parents* is my way of educating mothers and fathers, whether they are thinking about having a baby, are currently expecting, or are the proud parents of a newborn infant, to better prepare them to be the best kind of parents possible. I have deliberately chosen not to discuss specific illnesses and diseases, except for the common cold. Why? Simply because your job as a parent is not to diagnose or treat sickness—that is what doctors are trained and educated to do. Your job is to recognize and understand what is normal for your baby. You must learn about what to expect and when to expect it. To do this, you must have guidelines and specific information about what makes a baby normal and healthy. That is what this book is all about.

With this knowledge, you will be in a much better position to know when to call your doctor for help. And, equally important, you will know when to stop worrying about the wrong things so that you can relax and enjoy your baby. This is what good parenting is all about. And this is the kind of parent you will become after reading this book.

You and Your Baby's Doctor

HOW TO PICK
YOUR BABY'S DOCTOR

"How can we find the right doctor for our new baby?"

There are no quick or simple answers to this important question. The best I can do is offer some suggestions and guidelines that will help.

Before I begin, however, I would like to note that I have chosen the pronoun "he" to refer to the physician throughout this book. As with the question of choosing a pronoun to describe your baby, the English language provides no graceful way to designate a person of either sex. Although there are many practicing physicians who are women, the majority of these professionals are men, and thus I have decided, with profound apologies to the women's movement, to use the masculine pronoun in my discussions.

During my close to twenty-five years of practicing pediatrics, I continue to be amazed by some of the strange and foolish reasons parents choose a particular doctor for their baby. One day, a new mother came into my office for the first time with her brand new infant girl. As part of taking a medical history, I always ask who referred the patient to me. Her answer was: "I met a lady in the supermarket wheeling her little baby around, and I asked her to give me the name of her pediatrician." In questioning the woman a bit further, she also admitted that she had never seen that woman before or since. Taking the word of a total stranger is a pretty risky way to pick a doctor—a decision involving the health and well-being of the most precious possession you will ever have.

One common mistake people make in selecting a doctor is to be overly impressed by affluence and to equate obvious signs of wealth with the competence and skill of the physician. Frequently nothing could be further from the truth. A flashy new car or a fancy, expensively appointed office does not mean a thing. When picking a physician, remember that there need not be a correlation between the size of a doctor's automobile and the degree of his expertise. I remember overhearing a bit of a conversation in a restaurant once. A lady whose voice was filled with pride was saying to her friend: "My doctor drives a brand new Lincoln Continental—he must be a very fine physician." Financial success and competence do not necessarily go hand in hand. Please remember that doctors are just as human as anybody else, with different tastes, values, and needs. The doctor who chooses to drive a Volkswagen instead of a Cadillac has his reasons, and these reasons have nothing to do with how good a doctor he is. Obviously, there are more sensible ways of selecting a physician, and I will discuss these as we go along.

Let me begin by stating some basic facts. There are many rural areas in our country where there is no problem in selecting a doctor. These communities have only one physician to service all their medical needs, and so there is no choice. Of necessity this single physician becomes your baby's doctor, and that's that. But in larger towns and in cities there is a choice to be made, and this chapter will deal with that problem.

Until very recently, almost all the babies born in the

United States were delivered either by an obstetrician or by a family physician. Nowadays, nurse-midwifery is a new option that has opened up for obstetrical care. The nurse-midwife is a registered nurse who has taken additional training in the management and care of mothers throughout the pregnancy and delivery. They are hospital-based and deliver the babies within the framework of the hospital's department of obstetrics. They work in association with an obstetrician who can be called upon if any complications or problems arise.

The family physician who does obstetrics (the old-fashioned general practitioner) takes care of the entire family and so has much experience in treating infants and children. He also knows you personally. Therefore, if you are going to be delivered or have been delivered by such a family physician and you have confidence in his ability, it makes good sense to continue with him as your baby's doctor. However, there is no law that requires you to do so. The choice is always yours. If you prefer that a pediatrician take care of your infant, go out and find one.

In the larger cities most babies are delivered by obstetricians, who are physicians who specialize in delivering babies and who have had a good deal of extra training. Since obstetricians (and nurse-midwives) do not take care of infants and children, a pediatrician must be found for the newborns they deliver. A pediatrician is a physician trained specifically and extensively in the diseases of infants and children.

One possible exception to this situation might be when you have been referred to an obstetrician by your family physician who does not do obstetrics, but who does take care of infants and children. But as a rule, women under the care of obstetricians need a pediatrician for the new baby.

If your town has only one pediatrician, then of course there is no choice. But larger towns and cities have many pediatricians. How then can you find the right one for your baby?

Most important is to obtain a referral from somebody you know and trust. One choice is to ask your obstetrician for a referral during your pregnancy. Very often he works with a pediatrician on the staff of his own hospital. This pediatrician will be notified when your baby is born, and he will examine her in the hospital nursery. In most cases, this is a good idea. The obstetrician and pediatrician can discuss any problems related to your pregnancy as they may affect the newborn. This discussion ought to take place well in advance of your delivery date. Early communication between obstetrician and pediatrician can be of enormous benefit to your newborn baby. Again, you must always remember that the final choice is still in your hands. It makes things much easier if the pediatrician selected during the pregnancy turns out to be the right one. Unfortunately, this is not always the case.

I believe that whenever possible it is useful for you to meet the prospective pediatrician before your baby is born. In my experience, this does not happen often enough, but it should. An appointment can easily be set up where a husband and wife visit the pediatrician during the pregnancy. Such a short conference can turn out to be most productive. In the first place, you find out where his office is located. This may at first glance not seem very important, but it is useful to know. If the office is located a great distance from your home, it can create problems for you later on. Second, you can get some idea of the pediatrician's "availability." Does he work by himself, does he have a partner, or is he part of a group? Can he be reached by phone for emergencies? No matter how competent the pediatrician may be, he is of little value to you if he or one of his pediatric associates cannot be reached in an emergency. Also, you can ask about his fee schedule. This is perfectly reasonable and you should not be embarrassed to ask. But most important, you will get an idea as to what kind of a person he is. Does he instill confidence in you? Are you comfortable talking to him? Or, on the other hand, does he turn you off? Does he act as if he is doing you a favor by talking to you? If so, he is not the right doctor for you or your baby.

This prenatal visit can also be helpful from the pediatrician's point of view. He has an opportunity to get acquainted with you and your husband, and he can answer any questions that may be worrying you about your baby. For example, should you breast-feed or bottle-feed? What supplies and equipment should you purchase? What effect might family illnesses have on your baby?

If the visit turns out favorably, you have gone a long way toward finding the right doctor. If it does not, then what do you do? You simply keep looking. Ask your obstetrician for another doctor. Ask good friends or neighbors with children of their own for a referral. Are they happy with their pediatrician? Is he supportive, interested, and available? Does he spend enough time with the baby, or does he rush his patients out of the office?

Another method of locating a pediatrician that is especially useful if you have recently moved into a new community and have no good neighbors or friends in the area to consult is to simply call the local hospital or medical society and explain your situation. They usually have listings of the pediatricians in your locale.

I'd like to now turn to a sensitive area of our discussion: how can you evaluate the competence of your prospective pediatrician? This can be a pretty tricky business and not easy to accomplish. Certainly a referral from another physician whom you know and trust can be very helpful. He will make every attempt to refer you to an equally competent physician. But what can you do when you are required to find a doctor on your own?

In such a case, there are two important questions that you are entitled to ask of the new doctor:

(1) What kind of professional training has he had in pediatrics? and (2) What are his hospital affiliations?

A physician who practices only pediatrics usually has

had a number of extra years of specialized training after he has completed his internship. This additional training is called a residency in pediatrics and requires a minimum of two additional years in a teaching hospital taking care of infants and children exclusively. After he has satisfactorily completed this training, he takes a special comprehensive examination given by the American Board of Pediatrics. This test is rigorous and difficult. If he passes he becomes a Board Certified pediatrician and then a Fellow of the American Academy of Pediatrics. He now can put some additional initials after his M.D., namely, F.A.A.P. Therefore, if your baby doctor has the initials F.A.A.P. after his M.D., you can be quite sure that he has been well trained. This is a useful piece of information as you go about looking for the right doctor for your baby. It is true that he may still turn out to be completely unsuitable for your needs, but at least he has had the proper amount of training and experience in pediatrics.

This is not to say that there are not many splendid and competent doctors practicing excellent pediatrics without the extra initials after their names. But if a blind choice has to be made, I would advise the selection of a doctor with the F.A.A.P. The doctor's hospital affiliations are equally important. Is the doctor on the staff of an accredited hospital in the area? Is he on the staff of a teaching hospital in the area—a hospital that has a pediatric training program? If your baby becomes ill and she requires hospitalization, you want to be certain that your physician has privileges in a good hospital so that he can continue to take care of your baby, rather than having to refer the infant to another physician.

Let us now assume that you have made your choice of a pediatrician. You can expect that he will check your baby either in the hospital after delivery or after you bring the baby home from the hospital. If you have been fortunate enough to select the right doctor, you can relax in the knowledge that your baby's health needs are now in good hands. Should anything happen to your baby, you can readily and easily reach your doctor—as often or as seldom as necessary.

Sad to relate, there will be times when, despite the most careful planning, you still may have made the wrong choice. Perhaps you find you can't communicate adequately with your doctor, or you find he is never around when you need him. In this case, my best advice is to discuss the problem frankly with him.

It is wrong to just hope that a poor situation will improve by itself. Tell the doctor fully and completely what is bothering you. He should appreciate this honesty on your part. Most of the time, frank, open communication will clear the air and lead to a stronger patient-doctor relationship. But if there still is no improvement in your rapport with the doctor, it makes good sense to think about changing. There is no reason to feel guilty about it—such a change may be necessary. I do not for a moment advocate going from doctor to doctor at the drop of a hat; this practice really creates havoc. However, I do believe that you are not forever married to your doctor and you should not stay together unless you are happy and secure with the relationship.

After all is said and done, luck still plays some part in finding the right doctor for your baby. Nonetheless, following the advice I have given should improve the odds in arriving at the right decision for you. It is terribly important to select the best doctor possible for your baby. Following the suggestions I have outlined will improve your chances of doing so.

WHY THE MONTHLY VISIT?

A pediatrician is in the business of preventing disease and detecting problems as early as possible. The regular monthly visits during the first year of your baby's life allow the doctor to do his job most effectively. These trips to the doctor are among the best possible investments you can make toward the future well-being and health of your baby. My hope is that this chapter will convince you of the importance of these regularly scheduled appointments.

Many new parents simply do not realize why the regular checkups (known as "well baby" visits) are so necessary. This lack of understanding results in too many missed and cancelled appointments, which can lead to real trouble for your baby. In a short survey I recently conducted among a group of new parents, I asked why they thought the regular monthly checkups to the pediatrician were needed. The two most frequent answers were: (1) "I really don't know. My doctor just told me to do it," or (2) "That's when my baby gets his shots."

There is some validity to both answers, but as far as I

am concerned, these reasons are not the important ones. The real job of medicine is prevention and early detection, and that's why your baby should be examined regularly.

It is certainly true that your baby will receive immunizations against many childhood diseases during his visits to the physician. However, you really do not need a trained baby doctor for this. A nurse can give a shot just as well as a doctor. The point to remember is that an immunization is just a small part of the overall package of the office examination. Your doctor will examine your baby from top to bottom each time you come to his office. And why is this so important? Let me give you an example that should answer that question.

A six-month-old infant girl was brought in for her regular checkup. The baby was scheduled to receive a DPT (diphtheria/pertussis/tetanus) immunization that day. According to the mother, Yvonne was thriving, developing normally, and doing just beautifully. As I do with each and every child, I examined her from head to foot. Halfway down, in palpating her abdomen, I felt a very small, hard lump, perhaps the size of an olive, that did not belong there. It was early afternoon at the time. By 6:00 P.M. that same evening, the baby had already been operated upon, and the Wilms' tumor (a type of cancer of the kidney) had been surgically removed, along with the affected kidney. This is a very rare occurrence. It happened six years ago. Today Yvonne is completely cured and absolutely well. The diagnosis was made early enough so that this malignancy had no time to spread outside the kidney. It only takes one such case to dramatically hammer home the fact that the so-called "well baby" checkups are much more than what they sound like. Had this mother missed her appointment, the chances for this cure would have been markedly reduced!

Another case I will never forget further illustrates the theme of this chapter. A new patient brought in her three-week-old for the first time because of constipation. This was her third child. I asked her to undress the infant fully so that I could examine her. She was a little surprised since she thought that I would just check the baby's stomach and rectum. I started my examination as I always do, by looking at the baby's head—not her bottom. Lo and behold, her head appeared to be slightly enlarged in proportion to her chest. This turned out to be a symptom of a long and complicated problem. Briefly, this baby had beginning hydrocephalus (increased fluid in the head). She was operated on the next day, and, despite many ups and downs along the way, she is now fully grown and doing fine. Had the diagnosis been delayed for another month or two, there is no question that the results would not have been as good.

One of the most important functions of pediatric care is careful evaluation of the growth and development of the infant. Only by following the baby during the regular monthly visits can the doctor determine if, in fact, the baby's development is normal or not. A baby doctor is trained to pick up any deficits, however slight or subtle. It is extremely important that any lag in growth or development be diagnosed promptly so that appropriate treatment can be started as soon as possible.

Another important reason for the monthly visit is that parents have many questions about how to bring up their baby. These questions should be answered by the baby's doctor, not by some well-meaning friend or relative. I suggest to my patients that they bring along a written list. Your doctor will be happy to spend as much time as is necessary to answer any and all your questions.

Monthly visits during the first year also serve to establish an ongoing relationship between you and your baby's doctor. As a result of this relationship, not only do you learn about your baby, but your doctor learns about you. This is very important when it comes to asking for telephone advice. Your doctor can make a much more intelligent and meaningful decision if he knows your baby and knows how you think and function. I find it much more difficult to evaluate a problem on the phone from a parent I have not met. Again, an actual case can best illustrate this point. An old patient of mine had a new baby. In the past she had called me very seldom except when there was real trouble. Her judgment had been uniformly good, and she was extremely reliable. One morning she called me, quite apologetic, and reported that it was probably nothing but she did not like the way the baby was acting. "He just seems a little bit sluggish," she said. Knowing this lady quite well and respecting her judgment, I arranged for her to bring the baby right to the office. This infant turned out to have cretinism (nonfunctioning thyroid gland). After the appropriate tests confirmed the diagnosis, the child was placed on thyroid medication and has done remarkably well. He is now fifteen years old and is normal in every respect. If the diagnosis of cretinism had not been made early enough, permanent brain damage would have resulted.

Each and every pediatrician has his own list of dramatic stories illustrating the importance of early diagnosis and treatment. We also could tell about many other less dramatic situations in which early diagnosis and treatment was also important. An inguinal hernia must be diagnosed before it strangulates; a child with a mild iron deficiency anemia must be diagnosed before the anemia becomes so severe that it causes serious illness. I could list many more examples, but I think that I have made my point.

The subject of the need for periodic "well baby" checkups reminds me of one of my patients who gave birth in her automobile on the Long Island Expressway. She didn't have time to get to the hospital, and she was delivered by a policeman who arrived on the scene just in time. The baby was healthy and did fine. Why not conclude from this that policemen rather than obstetricians should deliver all babies? Obviously, this is ridiculous. Your obstetrician is your insurance policy that if there is any difficulty in the delivery, it will be handled skillfully. In the same way your pediatrician is your insurance policy that your new baby will get the best medical attention possible.

A final word. Make sure that you keep your appointments with your baby's doctor. These visits are critical to the future health of your infant. They go a long way toward allowing your doctor to do the job that he has been trained to do: the task of preventing disease and treating problems before they are too advanced to be manageable. There is no excuse for neglecting this crucial area of health care for your new baby.

WHEN TO CALL YOUR DOCTOR

The best one-sentence answer I can give to this large question is that you should report to your doctor any significant *change* in your baby's normal behavior. If your baby looks or acts differently from usual, your doctor must be notified. I cannot cover each and every possible reason for calling your physician. I will, however, give you the most important signs and symptoms requiring prompt action on your part.

1) **Color:** Caucasian babies are normally pink. If your baby becomes pale or develops a yellow discoloration of his skin or sclera (white of the eye), it is time to call the doctor.

2) **Breathing:** If you notice that your baby is breathing more rapidly than usual or is actually gasping for breath, report this to your doctor. A good tip to remember is to look at your baby's chest while she is breathing. If you notice that her chest is being sucked in with each breath ("retracting"), it may mean that there is a

lung infection which your doctor should be consulted about immediately.

3) **Cough:** All new babies cough occasionally. But if your baby develops a persistent cough, this must be reported. It often turns out to be nothing to worry about, but your baby's doctor should make this determination. (Incidentally, hiccuping and sneezing are considered normal, and you need not concern yourself with either.)

4) **Crying:** All babies cry, some more and some less. You will learn very quickly to recognize your baby's normal crying patterns. Babies cry when they are hungry, when they're thirsty, when they're lonely, or when they're gassy. If you notice that your baby is crying more than usual or if the sound of her cry seems different from usual, then you must call your doctor. A common cause of persistent crying in a baby is an earache, and she obviously cannot localize the area of pain for you. In such cases only an examination by your baby's doctor will determine the cause of the crying.

5) **Anterior fontanel** (the soft spot on top of your baby's head): Normally, the anterior fontanel is soft and flat. If you notice that it is bulging and tense, or if you notice that it is markedly sunken in, call your doctor. A bulging fontanel may indicate a serious infection such as meningitis. A sunken fontanel is found when a baby has lost too much fluid (dehydration).

6) **Irritability:** Some babies are placid and calm, while others, the so-called hyperirritable infants, fuss and fret a good part of each day. It will not take you much longer than one week to be able to categorize your new baby into one of these two groups. Should your baby become more irritable than usual, fussing and fretting for much longer periods of time, this may mean that your baby is sick, and your doctor should be informed.

7) **Appetite:** One of the best ways to decide whether or not your baby is sick is to watch the way she sucks her bottle or the breast. A normal infant has a vigorous sucking reflex. One of the first signs of something going

wrong is the weakening or loss of this reflex. If your baby becomes less interested in taking the bottle or breast, it may be an early sign of a developing sickness. Pick up the telephone and report this to your baby's doctor.

8) **Unusual drowsiness:** Each and every baby has a different sleeping pattern. Some babies sleep pretty much all the time between their feedings, while others are awake for many hours during the day and night. Very early on you will learn your baby's normal sleep pattern. If there is a marked change in this normal pattern (for example, if your baby had previously been awake a good many hours each day and suddenly starts to sleep all the time), this requires consultation with the doctor.

9) **Diarrhea:** By diarrhea I mean frequent and watery bowel movements. If your baby's stools become very watery, explosive, and more frequent than usual, this may mean an intestinal infection. In such cases it is time to call the doctor. It is important that the diarrhea be controlled before the baby becomes dehydrated (loses too much body fluid).

10) **Vomiting:** All babies spit up—some more, some less. If your baby vomits more than one consecutive feeding, especially if the vomiting is projectile (forceful) in character, this is a deviation from normal and requires a call to the doctor.

11) **Rashes:** All babies develop rashes around their diaper areas as well as some slight rashes around their necks and faces. These are not emergencies. On the other hand, if a baby develops any generalized rash over the body, if the rash is so severe that it causes weeping of the skin, or if there are actual lesions that seem to have pus in them, these conditions are not normal, and your doctor must be so informed.

12) **Constipation:** If, for example, your baby previously had been having four or five bowel movements a day and suddenly stops having any bowel movements for a day, a telephone call is required, since this is a marked deviation from your baby's normal pattern. On

the other hand, there are many babies who normally have one bowel movement every two or three days. If the constipation is associated with abdominal distention (swelling), it can be an emergency, and no time should be lost in notifying your physician about it.

13) **Urination:** Newborn babies urinate very frequently. In fact, their diapers are almost continually wet. If you notice that your baby's diaper remains dry for a long period of time, and especially if this is associated with poor milk and water intake, let your doctor know about it immediately.

14) **Fever:** If your baby is not acting normally and/or feels hot to the touch, take his temperature, using a rectal thermometer. Any temperature above 100° F means that your baby has a fever. Many times this fever is just due to not taking in enough fluids, to overdressing, or to keeping the house too warm. However, a temperature of 101° F or above may mean that the baby has an infection, and your doctor should be called.

15) **Convulsions:** Most convulsions that occur during the first few months of life are due to high fever ("febrile" convulsions). This is not so unusual a situation, and there is no reason to panic. Of course, your doctor should immediately be called. Rarely, the baby will have a convulsion without fever, and this may be more serious. Again, your doctor should be called, and the baby must be examined.

16) **Accidents:** If your baby suffers an injury to her head, especially if this injury is associated with loss of consciousness or with vomiting, your doctor should be notified immediately. If the baby is accidentally cut and there is a lot of bleeding, again, call the doctor. The bleeding area should be cleaned with an appropriate antiseptic, and steady pressure should be applied with a clean gauze pad or clean handkerchief. Some of these lacerations require suturing to close them. You must describe the size and depth of the cut to your doctor so that he may decide the proper course of action to take. If

your baby is accidentally burned by a hot liquid or a caustic agent, especially if the area of burn is large, do not take care of this by yourself. Call your doctor for advice.

17) **Poison:** If your baby accidentally swallows a number of aspirin tablets, for example, or if you find any other pill or liquid drug lying around your baby, there may be an emergency, and your doctor should be called at once.

18) **Loss of consciousness:** This is an obvious reason for immediate medical intervention.

When you call your doctor, it is important for you to have a pencil and paper with you at the telephone. When you speak to him, be specific.

Suppose your baby develops a fever. Tell your doctor the age of your baby, the actual temperature, the length of time the baby has had the fever, what symptoms you have been able to notice about your baby, and whether or not she has been exposed to anybody else with an illness during the past few days. Your doctor needs specific information in order to properly evaluate your baby's condition. Listen to his instructions and write down what he says.

Most illnesses are soon over and are no cause for worry. However, do not hesitate to call your doctor even when you can't explain to him why the baby is acting differently from usual. When in doubt, make the call. It's better to be overcautious than sorry later. Your baby can't tell you what is wrong. Don't wait until your baby is very sick before you call for help.

Here is another piece of advice. Real emergencies may occur at times when your baby's doctor is not immediately available. In such cases, take your baby to the nearest hospital emergency room. It makes good sense for you to find out ahead of time where this facility is located.

Your doctor will certainly appreciate knowing that there may be a problem *before* the baby becomes seriously ill. If it turns out that you are worrying needlessly, he will reassure you and you can rest easy. Your baby's doctor realizes that parents are often very inexperienced and that it takes time to develop judgment about what is important. So never feel guilty about calling your doctor, even if you think that your question might be foolish. Your doctor should be just as interested in the health and well-being of your baby as you are.

Any physician worth his salt should be sympathetic and supportive. If you do not find this to be the case, my advice is to discuss the situation with him. Tell him exactly what is bothering you and try to establish good, helpful communication. If you cannot work things out to your mutual satisfaction, I would suggest you look for another doctor for your baby.

IMMUNIZATIONS

Bacteria have existed since time began. Before the study of immunology gave us vaccines to protect against these terrible diseases, whole populations were wiped out by epidemics. The vaccines currently available are safe, easy to administer, and effective. Despite this, a large percentage of our children are still inadequately protected. In this day and age it is criminal not to make sure that each and every child is immunized against the diseases for which we have excellent protective vaccines.

The main purpose of this chapter is to remind you to get busy right now! You must make sure that your baby receives all the immunizations he requires. This means that he should be fully protected by the time he is two years old. There is no excuse for neglecting this very important area of health care.

Many of us still remember vividly the dreadful fear of smallpox and the horror of living through a polio epidemic. Nowadays, hardly anybody gives these killer diseases a second thought. In the 1970s a needle in the arm or rump or a few drops of a sugary liquid into the mouth, and presto—permanent protection against another vicious disease. With the widespread use of these vaccines, the incidence of measles and polio has decreased tremendously. As a result, too many of us have been lulled into a false sense of security. These dangerous and potentially lethal bugs are still around. If enough children are not given their immunizations, the chance of an epidemic reemerging increases. The sad fact is that currently over five million preschool children in the United States are not fully immunized and protected. One out of three preschoolers is inadequately protected against one or more diseases. This is a disgraceful situation and must be corrected as soon as possible.

An immunization is a safe and effective method that protects the body against certain diseases. The material that is given by injection or by mouth stimulates the body to produce substances called antibodies. The function of these antibodies is to fight off that particular disease whenever it attempts to invade the body. The protection that these antibodies produces is called immunity. After receiving the proper immunization, the child becomes protected against the disease for many years and often for life.

Each and every child should routinely be immunized against the following seven diseases, all of which can be very dangerous:

1) Polio
2) Diphtheria
3) Tetanus
4) Pertussis (whooping cough)
5) Measles
6) Rubella (German measles)
7) Mumps

Unfortunately, many parents wait until their child is ready to start school before starting the immunizations. A large number of children are, therefore, unprotected during the first four or five years of their lives, and this is just the period when they are most vulnerable to many of these illnesses. If an epidemic were ever to occur, they would be in very serious trouble. It makes no sense to wait until it's too late. Many parents are no longer concerned enough about inoculating their children, since there are now so few cases of the illnesses for which there are immunizations. It is true that the incidence of these diseases has decreased. But a very dangerous situation is developing around us. First of all, an attitude of complacency has resulted in more and more children's remaining unimmunized and unprotected. This increases the risk of an epidemic. As a matter of fact, there have been small outbreaks of measles in recent years in areas in which a large percentage of the children were not immunized. As I write this chapter, a beginning epidemic of measles is being reported in many states. There is also a further danger: there is now a reduced opportunity for unimmunized children to acquire their immunity by a mild or asymptomatic natural infection. It follows that these children are likely to grow up unprotected. Any infant born to one of these unprotected women is at great risk. These mothers will not be able to transfer any immunity to their newborns.

The effects of many of these diseases are most serious during the first few months of life, when the central nervous system is most vulnerable. Let's take for an example what happens with measles. If a pregnant woman has not had the measles vaccination or the natural disease, she will not be able to transmit any immunity to her unborn baby during her pregnancy, and the baby will be born unprotected against measles. An infant who gets measles can become seriously ill and may even die from it. A mother who has had the measles vaccine or the disease itself will naturally protect her new baby—and this protection lasts for about six months.

All segments of the population are not being

adequately immunized. Although the problem is greatest in the inner cities, urban ghettos, and among the rural poor, many thousands of middle-class children are also not being properly protected. A recent study reported in a pediatric journal clearly illustrates the scope of the problem. In checking over the records of a group of private pediatricians in Idaho, it was found that less than 40 percent of the doctors' regular patients were completely immunized by the age of two. Children taken to clinics had an even poorer record—only 22 percent were fully immunized.

At present, routine smallpox vaccination is no longer recommended. The last case of smallpox reported in the United States occurred in 1949. According to the latest information from the World Health Organization, smallpox has been almost completely eradicated all over the world. The last few cases have been reported in Africa and India. By the time you read this, it is likely that smallpox will no longer exist, except in our history books. Now there is a much greater risk from the possible complications of the smallpox vaccine than from contracting the disease. Therefore, both the U.S. Public Health Service and the Academy of Pediatrics recommend that smallpox vaccination no longer be carried out.

Most pediatricians start their immunization routine when the baby is two months old. The schedule suggested by the Academy of Pediatrics is the one followed by many physicians. There is room to deviate from these recommendations, and many doctors work out the routine that they find most efficient and effective for their purposes. The following, however, is the Academy of Pediatrics current immunization schedule:

2 Months	D.P.T.*	Trivalent Oral Polio
4 Months	D.P.T.	Trivalent Oral Polio
6 Months	D.P.T.	
1 Year	Tuberculin Test	
15 Months	M.M.R.†	

18 Months	D.P.T.	Trivalent Oral Polio
4-6 Years	D.P.T.	Trivalent Oral Polio

*Diphtheria, Pertussis, Tetanus
†Measles, Mumps, Rubella

The measles, mumps, and rubella vaccines may be given separately. If these are given when the baby is fifteen months old or older, permanent lifelong protection usually results, and no boosters are necessary. During the course of a measles outbreak or actual epidemic, the measles vaccine should be given any time after six months of age. Under these circumstances, a second inoculation of the vaccine is required after fifteen months of age.

Parents often ask me why it's so important to immunize their children against measles and German measles (rubella). They mistakenly believe that these are harmless illnesses that all children get sooner or later. The fact of the matter is that serious and even fatal complications can occur after any of these "simple" diseases. For example, encephalitis (inflammation of the brain) may follow measles and can cause permanent brain damage. If a pregnant woman gets rubella during the first three months of her pregnancy, there is a strong possibility that her newborn will be born with serious congenital malformations. That is why it is especially crucial that all girls receive the rubella vaccine before puberty. What I'm saying is that it is just as important to immunize your child against measles and rubella as it is to protect him against polio, diphtheria, and tetanus.

If a child is fully immunized against tetanus (meaning that he has received three D.P.T. shots followed by a fourth a year after the third), no boosters are needed for at least five years—even if he gets a puncture wound from a rusty nail. After the tetanus booster is given at about the time a child starts school, additional boosters should be given every ten years. If a child suffers a possibly contaminated wound and has not had a tetanus booster during the previous five years, a booster is required.

The tuberculin test is a screening skin test to determine if a child has ever been exposed to tuberculosis. It is not an immunization against tuberculosis. This test is repeated at varying intervals, depending on the risk of exposure and the prevalence of tuberculosis in your area.

There are some reactions which might occur following the various immunizations. Here is a list:

1) Polio: None.
2) D.P.T.: Occasionally some fever and/or crankiness, which starts a few hours after the injection and may last a day or so. On rare occasions, this fever may be quite high, and in such cases the baby's doctor should be notified. There may also be some redness and swelling at the site of the injection, which disappears in short order.
3) M.M.R.: In some cases fever develops between five and twelve days after the injection. At times, a rash also appears with the fever. This reaction may last a day or two and is no cause for concern.

You have to keep in mind that it is your responsibility to see that your baby is fully immunized by two years of age. The stakes are high, and there is no time to waste.

What to Expect as Your Baby Grows and Develops

THE FIRST MONTH

There is no question that a new baby will make many revolutionary changes in your life-style. Life at home now becomes an entirely new experience. Your new baby should bring a lot of joy and happiness into your house. She need not cause you extra tension and worry. Unfortunately, however, a good many new parents are totally unprepared and uninformed about what to really expect from their newborn. This lack of preparation results in tired and harassed mothers and fathers, leaving very little time or energy to really enjoy a new baby.

As a pediatrician with long experience, I know very well how important the first few months of a baby's life are in establishing a baby's behavior patterns and personality. Everybody agrees that infants flourish and thrive in relaxed and peaceful households, as do their parents. The purpose of this chapter is to tell you what your new baby is all about. This knowledge will make your job easier and much more pleasant.

Whether we like it or not a new baby is a lot of work.

There are many more new chores to be done. Obviously, this work load leaves less time for your former pre-infant activities. Nobody can do it all. In order to cope with the job at hand, you must establish a new order of priority. This requires planning and organization on your part. Cuddling and holding your baby, for example, is more important than cleaning the kitchen floor. Let some of the housework go—it is preferable to have a happy and contented infant than a freshly vacuumed rug.

I remember a new mother bringing her four-week-old girl into my office for the first time. Mrs. P had a huge grin on her face. "Dr. Eden, the past four weeks have been the happiest moments of my life. I enjoyed every minute with my baby. She is such a lovely little person and besides, taking care of Suzy gives me a terrific excuse for not having to clean the house."

Some behavior patterns you will observe in your infant are absolutely predictable. You can expect your new baby to startle frequently and cry a good deal of the time. She will grunt and grimace and squirm and kick. She will breathe noisily and irregularly. Your newborn can hear right from birth as well. Studies have demonstrated that newborns actually can see at birth, too, but they cannot focus effectively until about two weeks of age. By the time they are four weeks old they can focus on large objects and bright lights and can begin to follow them. During the first month a baby's eyes cross frequently, but this is no cause for concern.

Infants are strong and vigorous. They are small all right, but they are remarkably well engineered and well designed. They should be handled, held, fondled, and kissed, not just looked at. The more contact the better. Just remember that a baby's head is a bit wobbly for the first couple of months and should be supported when she's picked up or held.

Your new baby can be taken outside as long as the weather is reasonably good. I would suggest that you avoid crowds when you do take her out, however. There is no point in increasing the newborn's risk of exposure to illness.

Visitors to your house certainly should be welcome, but they should be cautioned not to cough or breathe all over the new baby. If they are allowed to do so, cold germs and other respiratory infections are spread to the baby very fast. If one of your guests insists on kissing your new addition, make sure it's not on the baby's mouth.

Your baby can be bathed any time after the umbilical cord has fallen off (this usually takes about a week). Until the cord comes off, give your baby sponge baths. A daily bath is not absolutely necessary, but most babies enjoy it. In any case, it's a good idea to bathe your baby frequently.

New mothers often assume that they must always stay close to their infants. This is just not so. Take some time for yourself. Get out of the house for an hour or an afternoon, just as long as you make arrangements to have a reliable substitute take care of the baby while you're gone. There is a whole world out there which you should take part in. Not only are these outings good for you, but in the long run they will be good for your baby. Even when you are at home, it isn't necessary to constantly hover over the baby, looking for trouble. The infant will let you know soon enough if she has any problems.

Many mothers are concerned over their baby's weight. Most newborns lose some weight while in the hospital nursery; they come home weighing less than they did at birth. By ten days of age they usually are back up to their original weight, however, and during the first month they gain an average of between one and one-and-a-half pounds. I do not recommend that you have an infant scale at home. The weighing and measuring of your baby can wait until the first monthly checkup at your doctor's office. During the first month the baby grows about one inch.

Another question I am often asked is if the new baby is getting enough milk. If she is content most of the time and gaining weight satisfactorily, then she is getting enough.

A normal baby's desire and capacity will take care of her individual needs. The new baby usually takes a feeding every three to four hours, for which I recommend a modified demand schedule. We'll talk about this in more detail in the chapter on feeding. If the baby is fussy or cries less than three hours after the last feeding, simply give her some water or a pacifier.

How about sleep? This question actually comes in two parts—how about your sleep and how about baby's sleep. With rare exceptions, you will be getting less uninterrupted sleep than you did before. This will, sooner or later, cause fatigue and increased irritability. But there is a simple remedy for this. Learn to lie down and rest during the day while the baby is sleeping. I know what you are thinking. What about cleaning the house and doing the laundry? You must learn to postpone some of these chores. It is much more important for your baby that you be refreshed and relaxed, rather than draggy and half asleep all the time.

During her first month of life a baby sleeps lightly and moves around a good deal while asleep. She is easily awakened and thus it is a good idea to keep the noise level down a bit while she sleeps. A mother complained to me that her two-week-old hardly ever slept during the day, and it was impossible for her to get her housework done. "I always wait for Barbara to fall asleep before cleaning the house. As soon as I turn on the vacuum cleaner, she wakes up screaming. What should I do?" The answer, of course, is to vacuum while the baby is awake.

Very few infants sleep through the night during the first four weeks. They usually wake up every three or four hours ready to be changed and fed. And there is no way of avoiding these feedings. My suggestion to you is that there is no law that requires Mamma to always be the night feeder. Poppa can also get into the act. What I advise is that some duties and chores be shared between mother and father.

If you had a quarter for every time your baby had a wet diaper, you would be wealthy in no time. Infants are almost continuously wet and this is normal. It would be unusual if your new baby remained dry for an entire day or an entire night, and your doctor should be notified if this happens. As for bowel movements, my best advice is not to count them. Some infants normally have one bowel movement every two or three days while others have a movement after every feeding. What is important is that the bowel movements be normal in consistency. They should not be too watery, nor should they contain blood or mucus. It is common for infants to strain and grunt with each bowel movement, and you need not worry or do anything about this either. Occasionally, if the grunting and straining becomes very severe, flexing your baby's legs will help her pass her stool. Any significant change in the normal pattern of urination or bowel movements should be reported to your doctor.

The amount of crying a baby does varies from baby to baby. Some hardly cry at all, while others are more irritable and cry a great deal of the time. But it's safe to say that all new babies do some crying, and it should be considered normal. Please remember that babies cry for reasons other than being hungry. Sometimes they are simply thirsty for water, or they are wet or gassy or just plain cranky without explanation. It takes some experience, but many parents can learn to differentiate among the various types of crying after a few weeks. I'd like to add at this point that the old wives' tale that if a boy is allowed to cry too hard he will get a hernia is utter nonsense.

Here is a list of some common situations that are all harmless and are bound to happen during the first month:

1) **Sneezing and hiccuping:** These noises occur frequently, and are considered normal and require no treatment.

2) **Mottling of the skin when the baby's clothes are removed:** This, too, is normal.

3) **Diaper rashes and heat rashes:** Very few babies get by the first month without one kind of rash or another. There is no reason for you to feel guilty if your baby develops a diaper rash. To help prevent rashes I advise you to keep the baby cool and comfortable and to change her wet and dirty diapers as promptly as possible.

4) **Mucus in the corners of the eyes and in the nose and wax in the ears:** All these conditions should be expected. I suggest that you clean all these areas very carefully without becoming too vigorous.

5) **Cradle cap in the scalp:** This is yellowish crusting commonly seen during the first month, and it is no cause for alarm.

With this information in mind, you should now have a fairly good idea of what to expect during the first month. We will discuss much of this material in greater detail in later chapters. If you are in doubt about something, or really worried about your baby's behavior, do not hesitate to call your doctor. However, learning the facts about the newest member of your family—what to expect and what not to expect—will give you a better chance to enjoy your first month with your baby to the fullest.

FEEDING

Mothers often ask me whether I prefer breast- or bottle-feeding. The question should not be what I prefer but what you, the mother, prefer. In the United States at the present time, one in three mothers breast-feeds her baby. Put another way, two out of three babies are bottle-fed. Strictly from the nutritional viewpoint, both groups do equally well. With the excellent and convenient ready-to-feed, prepared formulas available today, a bottle-fed baby receives pretty much the same milk as the breast-fed baby—a beautifully balanced diet of water, sugar, protein, and fat, plus minerals and vitamins.

I am always very pleased when a new mother is truly anxious to breast-feed her baby, and I encourage her to do so in every way. Breast-feeding is convenient and economical, plus there is no problem with contamination. The mother who anticipates the breast-feeding experience with joy and pleasure usually does fine. Human milk is ideally suited to a baby's needs. In addition, there is good evidence that breast milk contains antibodies that protect the baby against certain bacterial infections, especially those involving the gastrointestinal tract. Breast-feeding is also a most satisfying and fulfilling experience. It is the most pleasant, relaxed method for both mother and baby to enjoy the feedings. The warm, close interaction of mother and baby is very important for the baby's future emotional health. All babies love to be held close and cuddled by the person doing the feeding, and breast-feeding is a perfect method to accomplish this.

Problems arise when a mother breast-feeds her baby for the wrong reasons. In my experience, the mother who is pressured into it by outside influences (relatives, friends, mothers-in-law, etc.) is making a mistake to even start. The mother who breast-feeds because she has been made to feel guilty if she refuses does not do herself or her baby a bit of good. It seldom works out well, and in a short time the baby is switched over to the bottle. Let me give you a recent example from my practice that illustrates what happens.

A new mother of a two-week-old infant called, extremely upset and frightened. "Dr. Eden, I don't know what to do. I have been breast-feeding my baby, but he just cries all the time. I am sure he is not getting enough milk. I'm nervous and irritable all the time." After calming her down a bit, I was able to extract the full story. This young mother never had any real intention of breast-feeding her baby but was forced into it by feelings of guilt. Her mother-in-law had informed her in no uncertain terms that all the women of the family breast-fed their babies and that if she did not follow suit, it would embarrass the whole family. It was obvious that the sooner this ridiculous situation could be straightened out, the better. After pointing out to the mother what was happening, I was able to convince her that her baby would do much better if taken off the breast. We promptly switched the baby to a prepared formula. I then called Grandma and told her exactly what I thought about her tyrannical attitude. The baby has done just fine on the formula, and so has the mother.

I would strongly recommend that you do not start to breast-feed unless you are enthusiastic about it. There is no reason to feel guilty if you would rather not. If you have an inadequate supply of milk or nipples unsuited for nursing, you cannot breast feed. In such cases, your physician will decide the type of formula that is best for your baby. On the other hand, if you can and want to breast-feed, I would strongly encourage you to do so. It's the ideal way to feed a baby.

The key to successful feeding—whether by breast or by bottle—is to be relaxed about the whole thing. You should sit in a comfortable chair during the feeding and hold your baby cuddled in your arms. Never prop up the bottle and leave the baby. (Breast feeding mothers, of course, don't have this alternative.) Take your time; there is no hurry. Each feeding should last at least fifteen to thirty minutes to completely satisfy both the hunger and sucking needs of your infant.

How often should a baby be fed? I suppose the best answer I could give you is to tell you to feed as often as is necessary to satisfy your baby's hunger drive, and this obviously varies from baby to baby. I do not believe in rigidly adhering to an on-the-clock schedule. I would, however, advise waiting at least three hours between feedings in order to help establish a reasonable feeding schedule. If your baby is fussy and cries less than three hours after an adequate feeding, the chances are he is not hungry. Studies have shown that it takes at least three hours for the stomach to empty. Try a pacifier, or a bit of rocking, or a little water. A wet or dirty diaper may also be the cause of the fretfulness.

Babies will cry for a variety of reasons besides being hungry. He will cry if he is wet, gassy, irritable from teething, unhappy due to unsatisfied sucking needs, or just plain cranky. Some mothers automatically assume that all crying is due to hunger, so they are constantly and continually putting the bottle or breast into the baby's mouth. This leads to all sorts of problems. Overfeeding may start the infant on the road to obesity. A fat baby often ends up a fat adult. Besides, an obese baby is less healthy and more susceptible to respiratory infection and orthopedic problems. The longer a baby remains fat, the greater the chances that he will end up always having to fight the battle of obesity as an adult. For all these reasons please don't feed your baby every time he cries. Most mothers can easily learn to differentiate hunger crying from other types of crying.

I usually advise my mothers not to wake their babies during the night for a feeding. If he is sleeping he cannot be hungry, so why feed him? However, if your baby always wakes up hungry at 2 or 3 A.M., it is a good idea to offer him a bottle around 11 P.M. or before you go to bed, in the hope that it will hold him until the next morning. During the day, allow your baby to establish his own schedule—by waiting at least three hours between feedings and by waking him for a feeding if he is still sleeping five hours after the previous one (this seldom happens).

I object to ever putting the baby to sleep with the bottle propped in the crib or in his hands. This improper method of feeding may cause the baby to choke on the milk, and you won't be around to notice. Furthermore, it has been shown that putting the baby to sleep with the bottle causes pooling of the milk in the baby's mouth for long periods of time. If your baby has teeth, the acids produced by bacterial action on the milk can result in early dental decay.

How much milk should a baby take? There is considerable variation from baby to baby. The birth weight must be taken into consideration in this calculation. Obviously, a ten-pounder needs more milk than a five-pound baby. There is a good rule of thumb for the majority of newborns, which is 2 1/2 ounces of milk per pound per day. As an example, a six-pound baby would require fifteen ounces of milk each twenty-four hours. It has been calculated that a baby needs fifty calories per pound per day, and since each ounce of prepared formula contains twenty calories (as does breast milk), we arrive at the 2 1/2 ounces per pound per day.

I now come to what I consider the most important concept about milk feedings. You must remember that if given the opportunity, a normal baby takes as much milk as he requires. The baby will stop when he is full. You need not worry about underfeeding your baby. If offered his feeding, he will take all that he needs for normal growth and development. Appetite goes right along with growth—it's as simple as that.

Allow your baby to decide when to end the feeding. Bottle-fed babies are often encouraged to drain the last drop, whether they want it or not. As the famed nutritionist Dr. S.J. Foman points out, this practice leads to an artificial end point to the amount of food consumed. This sort of bottle-feeding may lead to overfeeding. On the other hand, the breast-fed infant usually nurses until satisfied and is less likely to be pressured into taking in more than he needs. Of course, if your baby completely refuses his milk feedings or takes only a small amount compared to what he was previously consuming, notify your doctor.

How long should a baby be kept on the breast or formula? For as long as possible, preferably for at least six months or longer. If you stop breast-feeding before six months for one reason or another, switch to a commercially available infant formula and not to whole milk. The Committee on Nutrition of the Academy of Pediatrics recently stated: "When breast-feeding is unsuccessful, inappropriate, or stopped early, infant formulas provide the best alternative for meeting nutritional needs during the first year." Infant formulas are quite comparable in their nutrient mix to breast milk, while regular milk is not. Milk contains a much higher concentration of both protein and salt than breast milk or formula. This may cause an increased strain to your infant's kidneys, which is not desirable. Further, there is some evidence that regular cow's milk can cause gastrointestinal bleeding, and this may result in producing iron-deficiency anemia. For these reasons I believe very strongly in the extended use of breast milk or infant formula. More and more parents have been switching their babies to regular milk by two or three months of age, and this practice should be stopped.

When should solid foods be introduced into the diet? I am flexible enough to realize that some babies require solid foods earlier than others. I also realize that the mother's attitude about food must be taken into consideration. A baby who consumes thirty or more ounces of milk each day and yells for more certainly will need solid foods sooner than a contented baby taking only twenty ounces. Some mothers just can't wait for the day to come when they can start spoon-feeding their babies. Other mothers couldn't care less about solids. In my experience, breast-feeding mothers usually are less frantic than bottle-feeders about adding solid foods to their babies' diets. It has been clearly shown that too early introduction of solids is another factor leading to childhood obesity. More often than not, the fat infant becomes the fat child, and the fat child becomes the fat adult. What should be understood from the nutritional standpoint is that there is no urgency to introducing solid foods during the first few months of life.

Most infants in the United States today receive some solid food before one month of age. I've had mothers call me asking me about adding a little cereal when the baby is a week old. This is ridiculous. All it will do is give the baby unneeded calories, protein, and salt. Despite what you or Grandma may believe, solids do not help your new infant sleep through the night. Introducing solids too early can cause colic, gastrointestinal upsets, food allergy, eczema, and an early conditioning to sweet or salty foods. I believe that solid foods should not be added to the diet until your baby is at least three months old.

The sequence I follow for the introduction of solids

varies, of course, from baby to baby. The following would be an average schedule.

AGE	TYPE OF FOOD	TIME
3-4 months	Precooked cereals, two times a day	Morning and evening
3-4 months	Strained single fruits, two times a day	Morning and evening
4-5 months	Strained vegetables	Lunch
5-6 months	Strained meats	Lunch
6-7 months	Egg yolk, strained, commercial, or home-cooked	Morning

It usually takes a few days of practice for a baby to learn to swallow from a spoon. Each new food should be started by giving the baby just one teaspoon the first day and gradually increasing each day. Wait at least three days between new foods in order to be certain that your baby tolerates what he is given. The signs of food intolerance to look for are vomiting, rashes, gassiness, and excessive crankiness.

I am pleased that one of the leading baby-food manufacturers has just removed the extra salt from all their baby foods and extra sugar from most. Their competitors are starting to do the same. Whether you make your own foods for your baby or use commercial products, do not add sugar or salt. Your baby should not become accustomed to foods that are too salty or too sweet. This approach can help prevent the subsequent development of high blood pressure, dental decay, and obesity.

After six months of age, "baby dinners," teething crackers, and single desserts may be added to the diet. These are usually followed by junior and table foods. At around six to seven months of age, so-called "finger foods" can be given, such as zweiback, teething biscuits, toast, and pieces of banana. The baby may manage to get a bit of these into his mouth on his own, but most of it ends up elsewhere. By nine months of age, many babies can handle pieces of cheese, a slice of apple, and scrambled eggs (well done, of course). Manipulation of finger foods gives the baby needed practice in spoon-feeding himself, which may be started at about one year of age.

Six months is about the right age to start offering sips of water or juice from a cup. Most babies rapidly learn to hold and handle a cup by themselves. Getting your baby used to the cup will also prepare him for weaning later on. I see no necessity to start orange juice until a baby is six or seven months old. Most younger infants just don't like the taste and they may also develop rashes or spit up. Nowadays babies do not require orange juice since they get all the vitamin C they need in a daily dose of multivitamin drops, which are recommended for all babies.

Some babies (especially prematures) require supplemental iron in their diets. Your physician will determine whether or not this is necessary. Most infants have enough iron stored up to prevent the development of iron-deficiency anemia as long as they are given solid foods starting not much later than four months of age. Excellent sources of iron include baby cereals which are iron-fortified, green vegetables, meats, and egg yolk. The baby who is on milk only (bottle or breast) for the first nine to twelve months of age may well develop iron-deficiency anemia.

Milk is considered the complete food for your baby, and it almost is. The only essential ingredient missing in milk is sufficient iron. With this in mind, I would counsel against giving any baby more than one quart of milk per day, in order to save some appetite and room for iron-containing solid foods. In order to prevent iron-deficiency anemia, many pediatricians believe that iron-fortified formulas should be given routinely to all newborns. The Committee on Nutrition of the Academy of Pediatrics has recommended that all newborns who are bottle-fed be placed on an iron-fortified formula for the first year of life. This practice would go a long way toward preventing iron-deficiency anemia. If your baby is bottle-fed, your doctor will decide whether you should use regular or iron-fortified formula.

The fact is that most babies are taken off formula and put onto whole milk by four to six months of age, just when they really require extra iron. In addition, a lot of six-month-olds no longer are given much iron-fortified cereal, another reason they may become anemic by twelve months of age. It is, therefore, very important to include iron-containing foods in your baby's diet during the first year. If you do so, you will avoid the iron-deficiency anemia problem.

Many mothers want to know whether they should give their baby the milk or solid food first at a feeding. It depends on your baby. Some refuse any solid foods after taking their milk, and these babies should be given their food first. Other babies have no preference and take whatever is given and are hungry enough to take both.

A simple method that I have found effective for many babies is to start the meal by giving a baby part of his bottle, follow with solid foods, and finish off the feeding with the remainder of the milk.

The right attitude about feeding your baby is the most important thing. It is seldom necessary to fight or coax a baby to eat. There should never be a mealtime contest between mother and baby. If he refuses to eat, it simply means that he is not hungry, and so be it. He will not starve. A normal baby's appetite parallels his growth, and he should *never* be forced to eat. Many babies' appetites for solid food are minimal during the first six to seven months. Toward the end of the first year, the baby increases his activity by creeping, pulling himself up, etc., and his appetite usually picks up then.

Mealtimes should be relaxed and unhurried. Feeding time should be happy and not a time of tension and frustration. Your baby's appetite should be the only factor in determining the amount of food he eats. Just offer him the right kinds of food. You probably will think he needs much more food than he actually requires. As I stated earlier, extra weight does not mean extra health, and a fat baby is not necessarily a healthy baby. Allow your baby to grow and gain at his own pace under your doctor's supervision, and you will never go wrong.

SLEEP

In my experience, I find that too few parents are prepared to accept their new baby's sleeping habits. Many mothers and fathers are unpleasantly surprised to find their own long-established sleep patterns are disrupted by their new baby. Instead of realizing that this is normal, they become overly concerned, upset, and angry, besides becoming very tired. This leads to the use of a bottle to quiet the baby every time she whimpers or fusses, and this is wrong. If it has been less than three hours since the last feeding, it is unlikely that your baby is crying because of hunger (since it takes at least three hours for the stomach to empty). Even worse, harrassed parents sometimes take the crying baby into their own bed during the night. This should never be done. Just accept the fact that it is normal for a young infant to sleep in short snatches and to make all sorts of noises while doing so. Learn your baby's sleep patterns and adjust accordingly. Let's consider, for example, a baby who is usually up for two separate feedings during the night and who sleeps for four hours each afternoon. It makes good sense for you to rest, too, during this nap period rather than spending that time cleaning the house. Nobody can be on the go day and night.

A relaxed approach to the sleep situation from the start is helpful. Parental tension does rub off on the baby. This results in an overly tense and irritable baby. Usually, relaxed parents produce relaxed babies, a theme that you will find repeated throughout this book.

There is another important reason for becoming familiar with your baby's sleep habits. It will make it easy for you to recognize any sudden changes in her sleep pattern that may mean that your infant is ill. In such cases, your baby's physician should be consulted.

How much sleep does the new baby need?

Each baby is different as far as the amount of sleep she requires. Your baby will sleep long enough to satisfy her particular needs; so there is no specific answer to the question in terms of hours and minutes. When your baby is tired enough, she will sleep. It is that simple. There is no relationship between the amount of sleep a baby gets and the maintenance of good health. Some of the healthiest babies I've taken care of have slept the least.

What is the usual sleep pattern of the newborn?

I'm sorry to say that most newborn babies do not sleep peacefully between their feedings. The expression "She slept like a baby" just isn't true during the first few months of life. The usual pattern is one of frequent short periods of sleep interrupted by crying and fussing. This happens both during the day and at night.

During these so-called nap periods, babies make all sorts of peculiar sounds—grunting, wheezing, gurgling, sucking, etc. These noises are perfectly normal and need not be cause for alarm. In addition, many babies almost continually toss and turn during their sleep periods. I clearly remember my own son's habit of continually scratching his fingers against his sheet during sleep. It caused the strangest sound, especially when the rest of the house was quiet. This light and restless sleep is the usual pattern for the first six to eight months. After eight months of age, most babies begin to sleep more deeply—more like adults do.

How long does a baby sleep during each twenty-four hour period?

Once again, there is no specific answer. An interesting hospital nursery study was carried out on a large number of normal, healthy newborns for the first seventy-two hours of life. The average number of hours of sleep per baby per twenty-four hours was sixteen-and-a-half hours. However, some of the babies slept a total of ten-and-a-half-hours, while others slept twenty-three hours. This investigation clearly demonstrated the tremendous differences among babies in the total amount of their daily sleep. The study also showed great differences in the "nap" sleep times from baby to baby.

As your baby grows older, her total daily sleep requirement decreases, while the length of each sleep period increases. During the first two to three months, the average length of each nap is three to four hours. It is true that occasionally you can get lucky. A new mother recently told me that her baby slept through the night from the day she brought her home from the hospital. This is the exception, not the rule.

Will noise in the house wake up the baby?

I remember making a house call to examine a five-day-old infant. I got there and saw a large sign on the door reading: "Please do not ring bell—baby sleeping." Following orders, I gently knocked on the door. There was no answer. It was impossible for anybody to hear the knocking because the baby was screaming so loudly inside.

It is ridiculous to whisper, tiptoe around, or watch

television with the sound turned down just because your baby is asleep. It makes much more sense to allow the baby to become accustomed to the usual noise level of your household. Obviously, some adjustments need to be made since the new baby does sleep rather lightly. You must remember that her appearance on the scene is no reason to completely disrupt and inconvenience the rest of the family.

When will my baby sleep through the night?
I am beginning to sound like a broken record, but the fact is that again there is no specific answer. There are wide, normal variations. Most babies will start to sleep through the night somewhere between three and six months of age. Some will do so earlier, and some much later. As parents, you have a little control over this aspect of your baby's development. Feeding your baby every three or four hours during the day may help her sleep longer at night. Do not wake your baby during the night for a feeding. If she is sleeping, she cannot be hungry, so why feed her? However, if your baby always wakes up hungry at 2 or 3 A.M., it might be a good idea to offer her a bottle at around 11 P.M. before you go to bed in the hope that this will help her sleep until a more civilized morning hour.

Is it harmful if my baby gets too little sleep?
As far as I am concerned, there is no such thing as too little sleep for your baby. Assuming that she is well and not awake because she is ill, she will get as much sleep as her body requires, and that's that. It is amazing how little sleep some babies need, but it is really not that surprising. After all, just think about an adult's experience. Some of us function just fine with as little as four hours per night, while others need eight or nine hours in order to be alert and awake the following day. Babies are no different.

In what position should my baby sleep?

It makes no difference. She can sleep on her back, on her stomach, or on her side. The position that she is most comfortable in is the position she should assume. Most babies prefer sleeping on their stomachs. It usually takes only a short time for you to determine which position your baby prefers. It is important that she sleep on a firm mattress and without a pillow.

Will feeding my baby solid foods help her sleep?

To this question I can finally give you a definite, straightforward answer. Absolutely not. Many parents mistakenly believe that solid foods will "fill the baby up" more efficiently than milk and will, therefore, allow the baby to sleep more soundly and for longer periods of time. This is just not so. Milk is what your baby needs, and milk is what will satisfy all her needs, at least for the first three months of life. Introducing solid foods too early may cause gastrointestinal symptoms such as vomiting, diarrhea, or constipation. As I mentioned, it also may predispose the baby to becoming obese. My best advice is not to start solid foods too early.

Should my baby sleep in a separate room?

If it is at all possible, I certainly would recommend it. As long as the baby is within hearing distance, a separate room is the ideal situation. There is absolutely no reason to hover over your baby continually. She will not choke or suffocate while sleeping.

What should the temperature of the baby's room be?

Babies are much more comfortable and sleep more soundly and more peacefully in a cool environment. Many parents have a tendency to overheat their babies' rooms. You should remember that your infant's temperature is the same as your own. A baby does not need more blankets or a warmer room than an adult. If you feel uncomfortable and warm so will your baby. I have yet to see a mother under-dress her baby or keep her room too cold. Open the windows and let some fresh air into the room—as long as you arrange it so that no draft blows directly on the baby.

What about air conditioning?

By all means, yes. Despite what Grandma may say, babies do not catch cold or pneumonia from air conditioning. Place the crib so that the cool air does not blow directly on the baby. She will sleep more soundly in a comfortable, cool room, and as a further bonus, the steady humming noise of the air conditioner can actually help put her to sleep.

Can I let my baby cry herself to sleep?

Yes, you can. Very often there comes a time when this may be the only way to help establish proper sleeping habits. At around three months of age, some babies who previously did not resist sleep begin to do so. Other cranky and colicky three-month-olds who have been held a lot and fussed with continue to fight sleep. The more these babies are rocked, held, or walked, the longer they cry. The best solution in these cases may be to allow the baby to cry herself to sleep. Simply walk out of the room and try not to listen. The crying will not hurt the baby even if it lasts a long time. (Crying, by the way, does not cause hernias.)

It is true that it is difficult to listen to your baby scream, but there are times when there is no choice. If you have the inner strength to get through two or three trying nights, the results will be well worth it. Your baby will begin going off to sleep much more rapidly and easily. In the long run, this is very beneficial. If these suggestions are followed, your baby will probably have a regular bedtime and sleep routine by the time she's six months old.

No, she won't sleep late on Sunday mornings, but that's a bit too much to expect, isn't it?

CRYING

All new babies cry. If you stop to think about it, this is a good thing. Since an infant can't talk, the only way he can communicate his needs to you is by crying. As a matter of fact, if a baby never cried, it would be something to worry about. As I tell new mothers and fathers, be happy if your baby has a loud and vigorous cry. This is one of the important signs pointing to a healthy, active infant.

Many expectant parents are convinced that they will not be able to find out why their babies cry. Take my word for it—in a matter of a week or two you will usually be able to recognize the different types of crying. Always remember that no two babies are alike. Each one has his own individual pattern of behavior, and crying is part of it.

Some infants cry more than others. The amount of crying is in no way related to the general health of the baby. The placid baby who rarely cries is no healthier than the more irritable baby who spends a good part of each day fretting and wailing.

Let's get down to some specifics. In my experience, the five most common causes of crying during the first few months of life are:

1) Fatigue
2) Hunger
3) Loneliness
4) Colic
5) Irritability

Let's discuss these causes one at a time.

1) **Fatigue:** This is a very common cause of crying during the first few months of life. Most parents do not think about this reason often enough. An over-tired baby, for whatever reason, becomes cranky and irritable. He fusses and cries and does not settle down until he has finally fallen asleep. Try rocking him or using a pacifier. Sometimes music or the sound of a vacuum cleaner will make him fall asleep. When he wakes up after a good sleep, he is less irritable and happier, unless, of course, he is hungry.

2) **Hunger:** This is certainly an important cause of crying. However, I think that too many parents assume that every time a baby cries it means he is hungry. This just is not so. There are many other reasons why a baby cries besides being hungry. One of the results of this automatic association of crying and hunger is overfeeding, and this can start your baby on the road to obesity. Take my word for it, it is not healthy for a baby to gain weight too rapidly during the first few months. If you pick up your baby and he stops crying, he certainly was not crying because he was hungry. It usually takes at least three hours for his stomach to empty; so it is unlikely that a baby will become hungry much before three hours has passed, provided his previous feeding was adequate.

3) **Loneliness:** Very frequently a new baby cries simply because he is lonely. If you pick the baby up and

hold him and he calms down and promptly stops crying, he was probably just plain lonely. You cannot "spoil" a baby during the first two or three months of life. So don't worry about picking up your lonely or tired baby when he is crying.

4) **Colic:** This is a subject unto itself and will be covered in a later chapter. Very briefly, colic is a condition in which a normal baby has a crying period each day, usually at the same time. This episode may last for hours. If you are unlucky, the colicky period will be during the middle of the night. The cause of colic is unknown, although there are many theories. If your baby has colic, your doctor may prescribe some medication to relieve the symptoms. But the key to recognizing colic is that you can just about set your watch by the time your baby starts crying each day. The crying of colic is loud, and the infant is obviously in pain.

5) **Irritability:** Some babies are just more irritable than others. We call this type of infant hypertonic. These babies are tense and jumpy and fussy. They are fretful and cry a good part of the time. This is their normal pattern of behavior (as opposed to that of the placid and calm babies who do very little crying). I have found that a pacifier helps these irritable infants calm down.

Hypertonic babies are not easy to live with. However, their parents should console themselves with the knowledge that their babies are not sick and that the irritability will gradually subside.

There are a number of less common causes of crying that you should be aware of. Among these are

1) **Wet or dirty diapers:** Some babies are quite fastidious and become very upset when their diaper is wet or dirty. Most babies couldn't care less. It is easy to learn the category into which your baby belongs. If your crying baby has a wet or dirty diaper, change it and see what happens. If the crying stops you know where you stand.

2) **Tight or restrictive clothing or blankets:** Many babies are upset when they are bound down too tightly and are much happier when looser clothing or blankets are used.

3) **Being stuck by a diaper pin:** It does not happen very often, but it should always be considered. My own son had it done to him by his pediatrician father. Just clean the affected area with an antiseptic, and try not to do it again. Or use a disposable diaper with paper tape.

4) **Being too warm and thirsty:** Most parents have a tendency to keep the house too warm. I rarely see a baby under-dressed or a house that is too cold. There is no reason to keep a house warmer than usual with the arrival of the new baby. Babies are uncomfortable when overheated and so they cry. Offering a bit of water and opening the windows does wonders to cut down this cause of crying.

5) **Illness:** Everybody worries about this. The question that is often asked of me is: "Will I be able to tell when my baby is crying because he is sick?" Most of the time you can. If he looks different or there is a change in his normal behavior pattern, he may be ill, and your doctor should be notified. If your baby starts coughing a great deal or develops vomiting or diarrhea, your doctor must be called. But if he is acting normally without any change in behavior, it is unlikely that he is crying because he is sick.

6) **Difficulty having a bowel movement:** Some babies cry lustily after a feeding because they cannot pass their stool. It may be necessary to use a suppository occasionally in such a situation. Putting some ointment around the anal opening also helps.

After all is said and done, we are still left with one more type of crying—unexplained episodes of crying. My best advice here is to learn to live with them. Crying in itself cannot hurt your baby, and as I frequently suggest to parents, think of it as just another form of exercise.

It is not unusual, by the way, for newborns to cry

without tears. Most babies manufacture tears by one month of age. However, it is not uncommon for tearing to be delayed somewhat beyond that age.

As I have said before, hernias in boys are *not* caused by crying. Let's put to rest once and for all this widely accepted old wives' tale. A hernia develops because of a congenital weakness in the inguinal area and for no other reason. If this weakness is present, the hernia will pop out sooner or later, whether or not the baby does a lot of crying. I remember seeing a new mother with her four-month-old boy. Mrs. P looked exhausted, as if she had not slept in weeks. In point of fact, she had been up a good part of every day and night since her baby was born, holding and feeding him. Why? Because she had been told that if she allowed Tom to cry too much he would surely get a hernia. Mrs. P never let him cry for a minute. What was worse, she kept feeding Tom every time he cried, and he was not only spoiled but was also getting much too fat. I explained the facts to this poor, tired mother. As she left, I thought to myself that the only hernia we would have to worry about would be the one Mamma would surely develop if she kept carrying her overweight baby around.

A final word of advice. If your baby starts crying, it does no harm to let him exercise his lungs for a few minutes, as long as you know that he is safe. It is hard to convince some new parents not to feel guilty when their babies cry. As we stated at the start of this chapter, all babies cry, and this is neither a reflection of the baby's health nor of the competence of the parents. Crying is your baby's way of communicating with you. With a little practice, you will learn to recognize why your baby is crying. Any sudden change in the degree or type of crying should alert you to the possibility that something may be wrong. In such cases, check with the baby's doctor. You must not become frightened or upset every time your infant cries. Crying is part of normal behavior. Relax and enjoy him, crying and all.

PACIFIERS

A favorite question new parents ask me is whether or not they should use a pacifier for their baby. The best answer I can give is "It depends." Some babies need a pacifier and some do not. It all depends on the temperament and sucking needs of the infant.

I'd like to start our discussion by putting to rest once and for all the notion that there is anything inherently wrong in using a pacifier. There really is nothing shameful or disgraceful about it. It is safe to say that many perfectly well adjusted children and adults walking around today started out in life by happily sucking on a pacifier.

It is somewhat surprising to me that so many new parents have strong negative feelings about pacifier use. Even more baffling is the fact that some physicians also object to it. This attitude recently was presented to me by one of my new mothers who said, "It just isn't natural. As a matter of fact, I would even prefer that my baby suck his thumb rather than the pacifier." I do not agree with this approach and I hope that after you read what I have to say, you will also develop a different attitude.

Seeing toddlers with their mouths plugged by a pacifier has probably led to the reluctance of many to start using one. I would agree that having your two-year-old walking around sucking away with a glazed, stupid expression on her face (especially when company arrives) can be embarrassing. Very often, outside pressures (from friends, relatives, neighbors, etc.) help instill guilt. How often have I heard grandma tell me: "My daughter never used the pacifier. Why should my grandchild use one? It's disgusting and harmful." If I cannot convince the doting grandmother that her attitude is wrong, I really do not worry too much about it—and you shouldn't either.

I carefully explain that times have changed and that the responsibility for the new baby rests with the parents and their physician. Since I am the baby's doctor, I expect the parents to accept my advice and suggestions. This approach may at first seem harsh, but often it is the only way to resolve the conflict and allow the parents to raise their baby without outside interference.

Many parents believe that if their baby uses a pacifier it somehow reflects badly on them. They believe that a pacifier is artificial and that if their infant accepts it, it must mean that the baby is unhappy and unloved due to inadequate efforts on their part. Nothing could be further from the truth. If it is true that the baby lacking in attention and affection is the one requiring the pacifier, it would logically follow that breast-fed babies would usually not need one. The fact is that just as many breast-fed babies require pacifiers as do bottle-fed babies. There is absolutely no reason to feel guilty about using a pacifier if your baby needs one. On the contrary, the sight of your baby vigorously and lustily sucking away on a pacifier should please you. You are providing your baby with extra sucking activity which she requires during the important first few months of life.

When a new baby is brought home, parents must keep an open mind about using a pacifier. Your baby's behavior pattern during the first few weeks will usually determine whether or not it is needed. Certainly your baby's physician should be consulted if you are uncertain. No decision need be made during the first few days. It takes a little while for you and the new baby to adjust to each other and for the new baby to establish her behavior patterns. After these few days, most newborn babies are either (1) calm, contented, and generally placid, or (2) fussy, irritable, with frequent crying periods.

In most cases, it is not difficult to recognize which group your baby falls into. Let me make it clear, however, that both types are equally healthy and intelligent.

If your baby belongs to group one (peaceful and quiet) and she cries mainly when she is hungry, she obviously does not need a pacifier and should not be given one. Her sucking needs are satisfied by her feedings, and that's that. But if your baby belongs to group two (fussy, cranky, and irritable), even after an adequate feeding, she is a candidate for the pacifier. Certainly a baby with full-blown colic also needs a pacifier to help relieve her discomfort. As I mentioned at the start, the crux of the problem relates to the sucking needs of the individual baby. The intensity of the sucking reflex varies from baby to baby. The so-called fussy baby probably has not had her sucking needs completely satisfied by the feedings (bottle or breast) and so this baby requires extra sucking. Withholding a pacifier from such a baby is unfair and a mistake.

Let's now assume that you have been able to decide that your baby requires a pacifier. The next important question to be answered is when to start using one. My best advice is to start just as soon as possible, usually when your baby is one or two weeks old. A baby's sucking needs are greatest during the first three months of life and then gradually decrease. Therefore, the pacifier is most useful early on. Give your baby all the sucking she wants and needs during this period by adequate bottle- or breast-feeding and the frequent use of the pacifier. During this first three months of life your baby has a very limited capacity to put her thumb or fingers into her mouth for the extra sucking, and this is another reason for using the pacifier early. If you find that your baby has not needed a pacifier by one month of age, she usually will not require one later on.

The next logical question to be answered is how the pacifier should be used. It should primarily be used to satisfy the sucking needs of your baby. Therefore, it should be used after feedings when the baby is fussy and cranky and unable to settle down. It may also be used between feedings during the fussy and cranky periods. A good idea is to remove the pacifier routinely when your baby has become drowsy and is about to fall asleep. A baby does not require any extra sucking while asleep. More important, pacifier removal before sleep prevents your baby from becoming overly dependent on it for falling asleep, and this will save both you and your baby a lot of wear and tear. Many babies accustomed to sleeping with the pacifier awaken each time it falls out and immediately scream, cry, and refuse to quiet down until they get it back. This process can repeat itself many times each night and, needless to say, leads to chronic fatigue and extra tension for all.

We next come to the question of when to stop using the pacifier. It has been my experience that most babies have less need for the pacifier by three to four months of age. Their sucking needs decrease around this time, and they usually become less enthusiastic about taking it. Many babies actually begin to reject it by spitting it out almost immediately. It is obvious that this is the proper time to start getting rid of it. But very often parents have become so dependent on the pacifier that they miss this opportunity to eliminate it. Instead, they continue to replace the pacifier even when the baby is no longer interested in it, and eventually it becomes a plug to keep the baby quiet. This use of the pacifier should be vigorously discouraged. The gradual elimination of the pacifier should, therefore, begin when the baby is three to four months old and should be completed within a few weeks. With rare exceptions, the pacifier should be thrown out before your baby is six months old.

Is there any harm in using the pacifier? If used sensibly and properly the answer is no. Pacifiers do not lead to future orthodontic trouble; almost everyone agrees that they do not cause problems related to displacement of teeth.

Check the pacifier to make sure that it is of solid one-piece construction and made of sturdy nontoxic materials. The shield must be firmly attached to the nipple so that the baby cannot choke on or swallow the nipple section (this has happened with poorly constructed pacifiers). Further, be certain that the shield is wide enough to make it impossible for it to get into the baby's mouth and that it has an easily grasped handle. As I mentioned, pacifiers do not lead to thumb sucking: on the contrary, my experience has been that pacifier babies seldom become thumb suckers. It appears that the extra sucking given during the first months of life often satisfies the sucking needs sufficiently to make future thumb sucking unnecessary.

Parents should never use a bottle of milk or juice as a pacifier. As the primary teeth erupt into the mouth, they will be exposed to a very acid environment for long periods of time and will be subject to extreme decay. We call this situation "nursing bottle syndrome."

To summarize briefly what I have tried to say about pacifiers, many babies are completely satisfied with the sucking they get during feedings (bottle or breast). These babies should not be given a pacifier. Other babies require extra sucking beyond their feedings and the use of a pacifier in these cases makes very good sense. Use a pacifier early and use it often but do not use it to induce sleep or while the baby is asleep. Do not use it as a plug every time your baby whimpers or cries. Plan to stop using the pacifier by three to four months of age, or a little beyond at the latest. Certainly, it should be long gone before your baby is six months old. There should be no guilt attached to the intelligent use of the pacifier. On the contrary, withholding it from a baby who needs one is wrong.

If my suggestions are followed, only good can come out of the experience. Your baby will have had her sucking needs completely satisfied, and, as a bonus, her chances of becoming a thumb sucker will be reduced. Your "fussy" baby will become less fussy, and the entire house will be more relaxed and in a much better position to enjoy the baby right from the start.

THUMB SUCKING

I consider thumb sucking in a child up to the age of four perfectly normal and harmless. The less you do about it the better off your baby will be. This is a subject of considerable concern to many new parents, and I hope that I will be able to put to rest the needless guilt feelings and strange ideas many parents associate with it.

During the first few months of life the only method your baby has to obtain food and water is through his sucking reflex. This ability to suck vigorously on the bottle or breast enables the baby to grow and develop normally right from the start. As a matter of fact, often one of the first signs of illness in the newborn can be the refusal to suck properly. In addition, this normal infant feeding mechanism gives your baby a sense of security and comfort. With these facts in mind, it should be a great source of satisfaction for you to watch your baby noisily sucking away on the bottle or breast.

In my experience, I find most babies begin some extra sucking (besides their regular feedings) by three months of age. They manage this by finding their fingers, especially their thumbs. This additional sucking on the fingers or thumb does not mean that your baby is hungry. Many babies can polish off an eight-ounce bottle of milk and then immediately pop their thumbs into their mouths and continue to suck away happily. These babies are obviously no longer hungry; so the thumb sucking they do satisfies a different drive. It is clear that babies just *enjoy* sucking. It is also clear that there are individual differences in the sucking needs of each baby. We don't know why, but some babies require more sucking than others. The babies with greater sucking drives become thumb suckers.

There are those who believe that thumb sucking is caused by teething, theorizing that the thumb sucking most often begins as an indication that a baby is feeling his teeth. I personally do not subscribe to this idea because, in my experience, thumb sucking usually begins before the baby starts to teethe. It is true, however, that the teething process can increase the baby's chewing and biting efforts.

Your baby has two choices: he will either be a thumb sucker or a non-thumb sucker. Simply stated, the thumb sucker becomes one because of his need for extra sucking time beyond the bottle or breast, while the non-thumb sucker has his sucking needs completely satisfied by his feedings alone. Both groups are equally normal and healthy.

Many new mothers ask me what they can do to prevent their babies from developing the habit. My answer is that it really is not very important to try to do anything about it, since thumb sucking is perfectly harmless. I do advise that every attempt should be made to satisfy the sucking needs of the baby completely right from the beginning. By doing so the baby will certainly be happier and more content. As an extra bonus his chances of becoming a thumb sucker later will be somewhat reduced. The two best methods of making sure that your baby is given all the sucking he rightfully needs are: (1) the length of each feeding, and (2) the intelligent use of a pacifier.

1) **Length of individual feeding:** If a baby spends too little time taking his feeding, he will more often require extra sucking after the feeding, and any intelligent baby finds his thumb splendid for this purpose. Some bottle-fed babies may finish their feeding in ten minutes or less, and this usually is an insufficient length of time to satisfy sucking needs. These babies are no longer hungry but still require additional gratification via extra sucking time. I would, therefore, advise that a bottle feeding take at least fifteen to twenty minutes. This may require changing the type of nipple used to slow down the rate of flow. I think it is important that a baby do a little work while sucking and not simply have the milk pour down his throat.

In the case of the breast-fed baby, the length of time of the individual feeding is less of a problem. It is very easy to keep your baby at your breast for about twenty minutes each feeding. In this way you can be reasonably sure that your baby has had both his hunger and sucking needs completely satisfied.

2) **Intelligent use of the pacifier:** If, after an adequate feeding (both in quantity and length of time) your baby still is fussy and cranky and can't seem to settle down, the use of a pacifier is quite helpful. (see previous chapter). If the pacifier is used intelligently during the first few months of life, you not only have a happier, more contented baby, but you will decrease the chance of the baby's becoming a thumb sucker later on.

Up to this point, we have been discussing the early, basic sucking needs of your baby. These basic sucking needs are pretty well completed by six months of age. But the fact is that many babies continue to suck their thumbs beyond six months of age—even some who have been given long feedings and pacifiers. Why is this? Simply because it gives pleasure and comfort to the baby who has learned to do it. The thumb sucking has become a habit, and a pleasurable habit at that, and so these babies continue to suck their thumbs.

Many babies do not bother with their thumbs during happy situations but pop their thumbs into their mouths immediately at any slight frustration or when they are tired. My best advice is to do nothing about it, at least not until your baby is two years old. Statistically, most babies will eliminate thumb sucking on their own by their second birthday.

Your thumb sucking baby has plenty of company, by the way! At least 50 percent of all babies suck their fingers or thumbs during this period. It certainly does not mean that your baby is unhappy, unloved, or neglected. On the contrary, it means that he has found an efficient, harmless method of enjoying life.

As I said before, most thumb sucking begins by three months of age and most often spontaneously stops by two years of age. But many babies continue to suck their thumbs to age three or four or beyond. These babies often revert to their thumbs just before and during sleep. There is still nothing to worry about.

We started our discussion by stating that thumb sucking is not harmful, and I should like to emphasize this point again. However, there are two exceptions, and one of them often leads to the other: (1) parental attitude and (2) thumb sucking after four years of age.

1) **Parental attitude:** Real harm can be done if parents have the wrong attitude about thumb sucking. *Never* chastise or punish your child because he sucks his thumb. You must accept the fact that this is normal behavior, and so it makes absolutely no sense to censure or shame your child about it. If you do, it can lead to real psychological harm. It is also important not to call undue attention to the habit. My experience tells me that parents who do not worry about thumb sucking rarely end up with a child who continues the habit past three years of age. Under no circumstances should restraints be used (such as mittens, adhesive tape, tying down arms, bitter

tasting substances, etc.). These cruel methods will really cause problems for your child, and besides, more often than not they just don't work. In fact, these vigorous attempts at breaking the habit can result in the actual strengthening of the habit so that these children can become the real "problem" thumb suckers who continue well into their school years.

If you have a child who continues to suck his thumb beyond the age of two, the best way to handle it is to talk to the child calmly, gently, without anger and without demanding perfection. Tell your child that he is getting older and that it would make you very happy if he would stop doing it. Often a reward system works out well. But the important thing is not to instill guilt—the child should not be made to feel ashamed. A positive, encouraging approach almost always does the trick.

2) **Thumb sucking after four years of age:** If your child continues to suck his thumb beyond four years of age, there is a possibility that his permanent teeth will be damaged. There are no hard and fast rules about this. It obviously depends on the length of time he sucks each day as well as the position and pressure of the thumb in the mouth. The permanent alignment of the adult teeth can be affected by a thumb sucker who continues after his fourth birthday, and this may require orthodontic treatment later on. But many late thumb suckers are lucky and do not need dental intervention.

There is general agreement among dentists that if thumb sucking is pretty well over by age four, there will be no damage to the adult teeth. Thumb sucking up to age four may affect the alignment of the baby teeth. The baby upper front teeth can be pushed forward and the lower teeth backward, but the movement of the baby teeth will not affect the structure or placement of his permanent teeth—which usually start coming out at about six years of age. I would strongly suggest that if your child continues to suck his thumb after he is four years old, you should discuss it with his physician. If he so advises, also discuss it with your child's dentist. Steps may be instituted by him to help prevent future dental problems.

There is another group of children, relatively few in number, who continue thumb sucking, occasionally well into their teens (almost always in their sleep). Most of these preadolescents and adolescents have no accompanying deep-seated psychological problems, and eventually the habit is completely eliminated.

Let me summarize these observations.

1) During the first six months, the basic sucking needs vary from baby to baby.

2) These sucking needs are best satisfied by longer feedings (at least fifteen to twenty minutes) and in selected cases, by the use of the pacifier.

3) The incidence of thumb sucking can be reduced but not eliminated by satisfying these basic sucking needs during the first six months of life.

4) Thumb sucking is common and harmless and serves as a great source of pleasure and comfort to your baby.

5) No attempt should be made to forcibly prevent your baby from thumb sucking, nor to shame or chastise him about it.

6) Thumb sucking usually stops without active intervention by the parents before four years of age, and in these cases there can be no damage to the permanent teeth.

7) Parental attitude is the key. You should not be overly concerned nor worried about thumb sucking.

I should like to offer one of my favorite pieces of advice: Relax and enjoy your child—thumb in mouth and all.

TEETHING

There is probably no subject more confusing to new parents than teething. I might add that there are times when the doctor is also hard-pressed to differentiate teething from other causes of excessive crankiness or crying (especially when he has to do so over the telephone). I hope this discussion will help you to better understand and cope with this problem.

Teething simply means the process by which the teeth push through the gums. What is puzzling to all is the great differences in the signs and symptoms associated with teething seen from baby to baby. Some have very little difficulty acquiring their set of baby teeth, while others suffer a great deal with every single new tooth. Nobody to date, including me, has been able to satisfactorily explain why this is so. Suffice to say, each baby's response to teething is different. I remember very clearly a set of identical twins. One of the girls never had a day's pain or discomfort as her teeth erupted. Her twin sister cried and fussed and drooled month after month as each tooth slowly and painfully pushed through her swollen gums.

When does teething begin? Again, there is much variation from baby to baby. Occasionally, a baby may actually be born with one or two lower central teeth. Some babies celebrate their first birthday with a mouthful of gums and no teeth. On the average, most babies start to teethe at about three or four months of age, and the first two teeth come in at around six or seven months of age. Before going any further, let me assure you that there is absolutely no correlation between the age the teeth erupt and the overall development of the baby.

Delayed eruption of teeth is *not* related to retarded development or decreased intelligence. Nor is it related to poor nutrition or vitamin deficiency. In fact, it makes no difference at all how old your baby may be when she gets her teeth. Furthermore, every baby is eventually guaranteed a full set of twenty baby ("deciduous") teeth.

What about the sequence of the appearance of the baby teeth? In other words, what is the normal order that they come in? Again, there is some variation and if your baby does not follow the usual pattern, there is no need to be concerned. The usual order of events is as follows:
(1) two lower central incisors (6-7 months);

(2) four upper incisors (7-12 months).

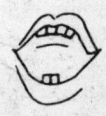

The two central upper teeth often come in widely separated. This is normal. As the rest of the baby teeth come in, this space gradually closes up.

So by one year of age your baby usually has six teeth— two lower and four upper incisors (the front teeth with

sharp cutting edges). Then there is usually a pause for a few months followed by the
(3) two remaining
lower incisors and the
four first molars (14-16 months).

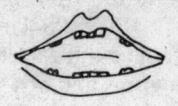

A space is left between the central teeth and the four molars. Next to come in are
(4) four canines
(the pointed back teeth)
(18-21 months).

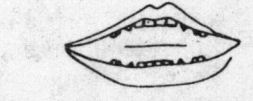

By two years of age your baby will probably have sixteen baby teeth. Finally,
(5) four second molars,
so-called two-year molars
(24-30 months).

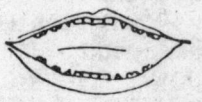

With rare exceptions, your child will have her full set of twenty baby teeth before her third birthday.

How can you decide whether or not your baby is teething? The first clear sign of teething is excessive drooling and dribbling, and this usually begins at about three to four months of age. Together with this drooling, some babies become quite irritable and may have a decrease in their appetites. Because of the swallowing of excessive amounts of saliva during this period, some babies also spit up or vomit more frequently than usual. Also, because of the swallowing of saliva, a number of babies produce slimy, loose bowel movements. Rashes may develop around the chin because of the extra drooling and around the anus because of these loose stools. Another group of teething babies develops coughs, especially at night. This night cough is caused by saliva dripping back into the throat during sleep. Still other teethers become fretful and cranky and often wake up crying at night.

Experienced mothers can often predict when a new tooth is starting to erupt by their baby's behavior pattern. Some babies, for example, have signs of an upper respiratory infection (cold) before each tooth; others develop diarrhea, get rashes, or start vomiting, etc.

I am often asked to predict when the baby's next tooth will appear. Let me tell you that it's not that easy. I remember what happened the last time I tried. After carefully examining the gums of a six-month-old, I told Mamma that there was no sign of any teeth yet. The next morning she called to report that during the night two teeth had popped through.

How can you be sure that the signs and symptoms your baby shows are caused by teeth and not by something else? It is very easy to blame everything that goes wrong on the teeth. Since the teething process usually continues for over two years and the signs and symptoms of teething are so variable, almost anything unusual that occurs can be attributed to teething. All I can say is that if you are ever in doubt, consult your baby's physician.

Let me tell you a story to prove this point. I remember a nine-month-old baby girl named Beth. Her mother called me one evening, apologizing for disturbing my dinner and explaining that the baby was screaming continually despite all the methods that usually relieved her teething. Her temperature was 103°. Beth's mother went on to tell me that she knew that teething caused fever, and so she wasn't too worried about that. She just wanted to know what else she could do to stop the crying. I arranged to see the baby that evening and found a severely infected ear.

The commonly accepted old wives' tale that teething causes fever is just not true! If your baby has a temperature of over 101°, it is *not* due to teething. There must be another explanation for the fever. What I have found is that the teething process somehow seems to lower the baby's resistance so that he becomes more susceptible to infection. The loss of sleep and decreased fluid and food intake during teething probably explain this lowering of the baby's resistance.

Faced with a baby who is having difficulty teething, what can you do to relieve the baby's discomfort? First of all, let the baby chew on a rubber teething ring, hard roll or teething pretzel, etc. A teething baby really appreciates the opportunity to bite and chew. Rubbing her gums with your fingers or with one of the commercial preparations that contain a mild local anesthetic can also help. If your baby develops a night cough as part of her teething process, elevating her head in the crib can be effective. For the occasional baby who is so cranky that she just can't get off to sleep, I recommend that you feed the baby the following mixture:

1 teaspoon whiskey
2 tablespoons water
1/4 teaspoon sugar

I recall being awakened one 2 A.M. by a frantic mother who wanted to know what to do with her teething baby. She asked about the whiskey, sugar, and water mixture on her instruction sheet and whether she should use Scotch or Rye! Any kind of liquor will do.

In researching this article I came across a very old remedy for teething that makes good sense to me, as follows:

Pour 2 ounces of gin into a wide-mouthed glass,
Dip the tip of your little finger in the glass,
Shake off the excess and rub baby's gums—then,
Drink the rest of the gin yourself.

Here is a summary of my thoughts about teething:

1) All babies teethe, and all babies end up with twenty teeth.
2) The age at which the teeth appear is not related to development or intelligence.
3) The signs and symptoms of teething vary from baby to baby.
4) The main signs of teething are drooling and irritability.
5) Teething does *not* cause high fever.
6) The best treatment is allowing the baby to chew and rubbing the inflamed gums.
7) It is much too easy to blame everything on teething. Therefore,
8) When in doubt, consult your baby's physician.

ACCIDENT PREVENTION

More children die from accidents than from all five of the most frequent illnesses causing childhood death put together. Not enough of us realize that accidents don't "just happen." *They are caused.* Nine out of every ten accidents to children could be avoided if parents were better informed about childhood safety. The key word is "prevention." Common sense, awareness, and some basic knowledge are all that are required.

The need for safety education starts before the baby is born. However, its greatest need is when a baby is between three and twelve months old. This period corresponds to the first phases of a baby's independent physical activity. This is the time when he starts to roll over, sit up, crawl, stand and begins to explore the world. Among all childhood accidents, infants have the highest mortality rate, and most of their accidents tend to occur between three and twelve months of age.

It is not possible to review each and every way a baby

may accidentally be hurt. The most common and important causes are:

1) Poisoning
2) Burns
3) Cuts and abrasions
4) Automobile accidents

1) **Poisoning:** It is estimated that 50 percent of all accidents to infants and children are due to the swallowing of poisonous substances. National Institute of Health statistics show that close to one million children under five ingest household products each year. As a baby begins to crawl and walk, he becomes a fast and fearless explorer, and just about everything he grabs hold of goes right into his mouth. The great majority of poisonings occur in the home. The most commonly ingested poisons are medicines, especially aspirin, and household cleaning products. The list of products that may poison a youngster is endless. The following eight make up a large majority of all poisonings and must always be kept out of the reach of your baby:

1) Insecticides
2) Laundry bleach
3) Kerosene
4) Medicines, especially aspirin and barbiturates
5) Turpentine
6) Furniture polish
7) Cosmetics
8) Rubbing alcohol

I remember making a house call to see a ten-month-old baby with a high fever. I was horrified to find the baby on the kitchen table with a bottle of aspirin and a bottle of rubbing alcohol right next to him. What was even worse, there was no cap or cover on either. I spent fifteen minutes lecturing the parents about accident prevention.

There are a few simple rules that have to be followed to prevent accidental poisoning:

1) Store all medicines in a locked cabinet or on a very high shelf.
2) Throw out old, unused medicine.
3) Never give your baby medication in a dark room.
4) Label all medication.
5) Don't keep cleaning aids under the sink.
6) Never leave babies unattended near medications or near potentially dangerous household products.

One of the most amazing statistics I have come across, and my own experience bears it out, is that there is a 50 percent recurrence rate in children who have been poisoned. In other words, one out of every two poison themselves a *second* time. This happens because the parents not only had not taken the proper precautions the first time but didn't learn anything from the first accident.

There is no such thing as a "universal antidote." The so-called "universal antidote" that is made up of a mixture of burnt toast, weak tea, and milk of magnesia (that all grandparents know about) just doesn't work. It is worthless and obsolete, so forget about it. The only true universal antidote to poisoning is prevention.

If your baby swallows something that may be poisonous, make him vomit immediately. The only exception to this rule is when your baby has ingested a petroleum product such as kerosene, or a lye product such as a drain cleaner. In such cases follow the instructions on the label, or give him some milk and immediately take him to the nearest hospital. If you go to the hospital, make sure to take the bottle or box of poison with you so that you can show it to the doctor in the emergency room.

If it is not a petroleum or lye product, make your baby vomit and call your doctor for further advice. The easiest way to get your baby to vomit is to use syrup of ipecac.

This is an excellent product that every household should always have around. Simply give the baby one tablespoon followed by some milk, and your baby will almost always vomit within a few minutes. If you do not have syrup of ipecac, give the baby some milk, hold him face down over your lap, put your finger or a blunt spoon handle down his throat. This should do the trick.

You should suspect that your baby may have been poisoned in the following situations:

1) If the baby is seen or found with an empty container
2) If he acts strangely, especially with stains or burns around his mouth
3) If there is vomiting, abdominal pain, drowsiness, rapid breathing, convulsions, or unconsciousness

In such cases, immediately call your doctor for advice. Poison control centers have been established in many cities, often associated with health departments. It would be very useful for you to find out if your community has such a poison control center. If it does, keep the telephone number available (and where your baby-sitter can also find it). These poison control centers have trained personnel who can answer your questions if your baby has swallowed some foreign substance. Giving them the specific name of the product as well as the quantity your baby swallowed will help them tell you what to do. About two thousand children die each year from swallowing materials found in their own homes. Anticipating the possibility of poisoning and safety-proofing your house will guarantee that you never will experience such a tragedy.

2) Burns: This is another common cause of childhood accidents and can be catastrophic. There are a number of rules related to the prevention of burns. Among these are

1) Keep the baby away from the stove.

2) Do not have any dangling electric cords in the house.

3) Keep your hot pans, especially of grease or oil, on the back of the stove.

4) Do not use overhanging tablecloths—these can easily be yanked down by the toddler. As a matter of fact, I recently had to care for a little girl who suffered a severe burn after pulling at the tablecloth and spilling a mug of boiling hot coffee all over her pretty face.

The treatment of the burn depends on its severity and the area of skin burned. A minor burn involves a small area in which the skin is just reddened. This is called a first degree burn. In such cases, the immediate treatment is to use cold water on the burn area for a few minutes in order to relieve the pain and then to cover it with a sterile gauze pad. I would suggest that you use a nonstick plastic-covered gauze since ordinary gauze may cling to the skin and be difficult to remove. If the burn area is blistered and small, treatment still consists of the use of cold water and then a sterile gauze pad. Do not disturb the blisters or use ointments. Notify your doctor as to the area of skin involved and what it looks like, and he will advise you about treatment. If the burn covers a large area, and especially if the skin is blistered or charred, cover it with a clean sheet or a thin plastic wrapping. Wrap your baby with blankets to keep him warm and take him right to the hospital. Do not apply butter or any salve or ointment. This is a medical emergency and it cannot wait.

3) **Cuts:** When the cut is slight, all that is necessary is to clean the area with soap and water and apply a sterile dressing such as a gauze square or adhesive Band-Aid. The use of a nonstick square is preferable. When the cut is deep, cover it with a clean bandage and call your doctor. These cuts may require suturing, and he will advise you accordingly. If the bleeding continues, cover it with a

clean gauze pad and apply steady pressure. Sometimes ten minutes of this type of pressure is needed to finally stop the bleeding. *Abrasions:* Babies fall a lot and sometimes these falls cause a rough scrape or abrasion. If the baby falls on a dirty surface, particles of dirt or small stones may be imbedded in the abrasion. If they can be seen, simply wash them off by gently cleaning the area with soap and water. If they are not removed at the time of the injury, the abrasion may heal over these particles and the baby's skin may look tattooed later on. Further, removing these foreign bodies later on is a more difficult procedure. If the particles cannot easily be washed off, the area can be scrubbed with a stiff brush. This certainly would be painful for the baby and should be done by your doctor, using a local anesthetic.

While on the subject of cuts and abrasions, I should like to remind you about tetanus (lockjaw). This is a very serious infection that is caused by a bacteria that may be found in a wound contaminated by dirt, rust, or manure. Puncture wounds are particularly prone to this type of infection. If your baby has been fully immunized against tetanus there is nothing to worry about. Check with your doctor to see if an additional tetanus injection is necessary. This is why it is a good idea for you to keep a record of all your baby's immunizations and the dates they were given.

4) **Automobile accidents:** This is an extremely important and neglected problem that you should be aware of. Since about one thousand children under five are killed each year while riding in automobiles and many thousands more are severely injured, there is no choice. Your small baby must be protected with a specially designed restraint. Holding your baby in your arms while riding in a car is not safe and the ordinary seat belt is also not suitable for a child younger than four. Your baby should be carried in a special automobile safety restraint beginning with his very first car ride, the drive home from

the hospital. There are a number of excellent commercially available infant carriers. They are all designed to face backward or sideways. The baby rides in a semiupright position secured with a harness. The carrier itself is held down with the automobile seat belt.

Automobile safety precautions must start when your child is born and must continue as he grows older. A child who is accustomed to riding restrained from an early age will continue to accept restriction. This will prevent a great number of serious automobile injuries and deaths. For further information related to automobile safety I would suggest that you write: Physicians for Automotive Safety, 50 Union Avenue, Irvington, N.J. 07011.

Dr. George Wheatley, the past president of the American Academy of Pediatrics and a pioneer in the field of accident prevention recently wrote a fine article on home accident prevention in *Pediatric Annals*. He lists six unbreakable rules for parents of babies. It doesn't pay to be flexible in this area. By following these few rigid rules, many accidents can be prevented.

1) Never leave your baby alone in the house.
2) Never leave him alone on anything from which he might fall.
3) Always keep the sides of the crib up when not attending the baby.
4) Always stay with your baby when he is in the tub. Even if he can sit up well, in a split second he might slip under the water.
5) Always keep tiny swallowable objects—pins, beads, buttons, and the like out of the baby's reach. No toy should be smaller than the baby's mouth.
6) Always keep medicines, aspirin, tranquilizers, cosmetics, poisons, and household cleansers well out of reach or, preferably, locked away.

The key to accident treatment is prevention. I have seen many tragic accidents happen through the years because home prevention techniques were not carried out. Don't wait until tomorrow when it may be too late. The time to start is *now*.

TOILET TRAINING

There is probably no other subject that causes new mothers more concern than toilet training. Too many mothers are frightened and worried about it, when, in fact, toilet training is a simple and normal developmental process that should not cause any problem. It is particularly interesting to me that I am often asked about toilet training at obviously inappropriate times; namely, too early, when the baby is less than six months old, or too late, when the child is already past three years of age. I remember one of my new mothers actually bringing up the subject during our discussion at the time of her baby's discharge from the hospital nursery.

I wish I could give you specific guidelines that always hold true, but this is not possible. Each baby is different, and there are no hard and fast rules that apply to all of them. But I can give you suggestions and advice that will be helpful in a majority of cases. By following these recommendations, successful toilet training can be achieved smoothly and peacefully without unduly

TOILET TRAINING

traumatizing either the baby or the parents.

Let us begin by spelling out what I mean by toilet training. This is the process by which you help your child achieve control of her excretory systems, namely, stool and urine. The emphasis will be on bowel control, since this usually results in the simultaneous control of urination.

You must understand that properly achieved toilet training is a great source of satisfaction and gratification for the child. You must also understand that very few babies train themselves—they need and deserve your help and guidance. I believe that an important factor in successful toilet training is the attitude of the child's parents. If you start with the proper attitude, the actual techniques are simple and effective.

What do I mean by the proper attitude? I can best explain this by giving you some historical facts. Thirty years ago most babies were toilet trained by one year of age. Coercive and rigid methods were usually employed. Unfortunately, these methods led to severe psychological problems in many of these children. In more recent years, the swing has been in the opposite direction, and today, many children have not begun to be trained by three years of age. Many parents—often the well-educated group—take this overly permissive attitude. They say, "Leave her alone, she'll train herself when she's ready." They believe that becoming actively involved in toilet training at any age leads to animosity, frustration, and friction later on. This group has misinterpreted the currently accepted pediatric approach of firm, gentle guidance to mean total permissiveness. I believe that the fear of ever frustrating your child is just as destructive to healthy personality development as was the unyielding and rigid superdisciplinary approach of thirty years ago.

The proper attitude toward toilet training (and, incidentally, toward just about everything else related to your child) lies somewhere between permissive noninvolvement and rigid overinvolvement. The proper attitude to strive for is one of friendliness, interest, and encouragement, along with consistency and perseverance. You will not frustrate your child by this approach to toilet training, nor will you allow the situation to get completely out of hand. On the contrary, a supportive attitude encourages your child to want to please you, and this certainly will be a strong influence in helping her master bowel control. If carried out this way, the toilet training experience will play an important part in forming positive traits in your child's character and personality. It will also build up a vital basic trust between you and your child.

There is a right time to begin the toilet training process, which varies from baby to baby. You will be amazed at how simple it is to recognize when the proper time comes. When your child is ready, she will need your help, support, and guidance. A firm yet gentle hand is the key to success.

During the first year of life, your baby has no voluntary control over his bowel movements and so they are completely irregular. Once in a while, a baby will be regular enough to catch on a potty before one year of age. Since this does not represent voluntary cooperation, but rather a conditioned reflex, the child is not really toilet trained. But if the child can do it without making a big fuss, go right ahead—it may help the actual toilet training later on. For all practical purposes, however, no actual efforts toward toilet training should be started until your baby is at least one year old.

Between twelve and eighteen months of age, most babies become aware of their bowel movements and are often very proud and possessive about them. A few babies may be ready to begin training at this age, but in my experience, most are not.

Eighteen months of age is usually a good time to get started. By then most babies begin to understand the meaning of praise, and they also start to become proud of their various accomplishments. There is some regularity to their bowel movements, but most important is the fact that the baby is finally aware of when her bowel movement is coming, and this is the crux of the matter. Starting at around eighteen months of age, you must try to learn to recognize the warning signals your baby gives before defecating. In most cases it is not difficult to do. Some babies turn red, others make straining noises, others squat, and still others suddenly stop playing for a few seconds. These signs are the key to the beginning of the toilet training adventure.

It is time now to bring out the potty chair. I prefer one that rests on the floor rather than one that is attached to a regular toilet seat. My reasons for this are (1) the baby has the security of having her feet on the floor rather than being frightened by sitting high above the ground; (2) the baby can use the potty chair by herself; and (3) this type of potty belongs exclusively to the child.

It is a good idea to let your child get used to her potty chair before actually sitting her on it for her bowel movement. This can be done by having her sit on the potty for a few days with her clothes on before the start of actual training.

Finally, the big day arrives. Your child, usually between eighteen and twenty-four months of age, is fairly regular with her bowel movements, gives you definite warning signs of a forthcoming bowel movement, and is familiar with her potty chair. Start to gently and firmly put her on her potty at the appropriate time. Be encouraging and optimistic. If nothing happens—and it usually will not for a while—don't get discouraged. Rome wasn't built in a day. When she is finally successful for the first time, make a big fuss about it. Say how proud and happy you are and what a big boy or girl he or she is. After proper wiping and cleaning, take her off the potty and give her a big hug and kiss. Be sure to put the potty away. It should not be used as a toy.

Patience is what is now needed. Very few babies are trained in a matter of days or even weeks. It usually takes months. Keep on putting her on the potty at the appropriate times. If she balks, continue anyway, even for a short period of time. Your child must be taught that you are serious and consistent about this business, so never give up for even a day. It will be much more difficult to start all over again if you do, and this inconsistency will create a lot of unnecessary confusion for the baby. *Never* chastise, yell, or punish your child when she is unsuccessful, and never shame her about it. Don't compete with your neighbor to see who trains his or her baby faster. Just be patient and encouraging, interested and concerned.

In the majority of cases, your child will be trained by age two to two and a half. When some success has been achieved, take her out of her diapers and put her in training pants during the day. If done properly, this can be a happy day for your child. She will be proud to be considered big enough to be taken out of diapers, and you should tell her over and over how happy you are about this achievement.

Some babies are just more difficult to train than others, and these children may not be trained by age two and a half or even by three. Despite your best efforts, nothing seems to work. Don't become frantic and don't feel guilty. Above all, don't make your baby feel guilty about it. There is nothing wrong with you or with your baby—nobody has to visit a psychiatrist. Sometimes putting the child on the potty for about ten minutes after each meal may do the trick. The important thing to remember is not to give up.

I have taken care of a great many children during my years of practicing pediatrics, and I have rarely seen a child who is not finally toilet trained by age four. If your youngster is still in diapers while eating her third birthday cake, don't get upset. She is normal. There is absolutely no relationship between late toilet training and lack of intelligence. She can still grow up to be a professor at MIT!

Just a few words about bladder training. As I stated earlier, successful bowel training often results in the simultaneous control of urination; so in many cases, it is not necessary to do much about urine training. A couple of suggestions may be helpful in achieving urine control: (1) wait for your child to be dry for about two hours, and then take her to the potty chair; (2) Use training pants. They help. The child around two years of age doesn't like her cold wet diaper, and this can act as a stimulus to more speedy training. Boys are usually slower than girls in establishing urine control. Just as with bowel movement training, there are many accidents until the child is two and a half to three years old. Don't worry about this. These accidents will stop sooner or later. Night bladder control comes last, and nothing should be done about it. Again, time will take care of it.

The most important points about toilet training are these. There is always some resistance. You will not stir up antagonism in your child by being definite and persistent in your approach. On the contrary, you will establish a strong positive bond with your child by helping her succeed. An interested, friendly, and encouraging attitude is essential. In most cases, eighteen months of age is a good time to start, but many children are not ready until about age two. Recognition of the warning signs of readiness for the bowel movement is most important. The process of toilet training should be looked upon as a natural event in your child's life and one of considerable importance to her normal development. She needs firm but gentle guidance. I believe that an overly permissive, nonparticipating attitude is just as bad for your baby as an overly rigid, tense approach. Common sense is all you need.

THE ROLE OF
THE NEW FATHER

Newborn babies are entitled to the intimate, loving care of both a mother and a father. But very often babies do not get it. Too many are being short-changed one parent. In this chapter, I will deal with the reasons why so many fathers are not sufficiently involved and why this situation is unhealthy. Based on my experience, I am convinced that, in general, the involvement of *both* parents in raising their baby is very important and pays excellent dividends later on.

Very often, fathers-to-be feel left out during the pregnancy, and their feelings during this time are sometimes the beginning of their attitude of noninvolvement. The pregnant woman is the celebrity, and everybody fusses over her every twinge, ache, and pain. The mother-to-be proudly talks about "her" baby and subconsciously starts to believe that the new baby is her exclusive possession. The fact is that we are all born with forty-six chromosomes—twenty-three of which come from the mother and twenty-three of which come from the father. In other words, Poppa contributes just as much as Mamma, and it would be well for all of us to always keep this in mind.

Many prospective fathers cannot help but resent the fuss and attention showered on the pregnant wife and "her" baby. The expectant father needs to be reminded (and must himself remember) that he is just as important in the overall scheme of a baby's growing up. This attitude will help reduce the strain pregnancy may place on the marriage. Further, the "our" baby attitude will set the stage for a father's positive, active participation in the upbringing of the baby right from the start.

Finally the big day arrives! The new baby is brought home. Again, the new father is often inadvertently forgotten.

Many mothers and fathers quickly fall into the trap of allowing themselves to believe that the mother is the only one able to really care for the baby. This can be the beginning of an unhealthy situation. The result is that too many children become overly dependent on their mothers, and too many mothers become overprotective toward their children. It is much healthier for the baby to have the love and attention of both parents beginning from Day One.

The arrival of a new baby drastically changes the ground rules in a house. The baby's needs come first now. For the parents there is much less uninterrupted sleep, less privacy, and many more chores to do. Many mothers take over the entire job of caring for the baby. In a short time they become harried and overly tired, devoting all their time to the new baby and having no time or strength left for their husbands or themselves. This situation obviously can lead to all sorts of trouble.

The first few months can be a most difficult time for everybody. Many mothers complain to me that their husbands are no longer as attentive and loving as they were before the baby was born and that the husband and wife are beginning to drift apart. Under these circumstances, a rift may be understandable. The father feels neglected, and he subconsciously blames the new baby.

A marriage that was good before the pregnancy should not deteriorate because of the new baby, but it sometimes does. A new baby should solidify and enhance a relationship. My experience has convinced me that the attitude of both parents toward their new baby is the key. When a father is made to feel that he is as important in bringing up the infant as the mother is, and that he is very much needed for this purpose, all goes well for the marriage and for the new addition. Mutual support and sharing is the start of real togetherness.

Given half a chance, most fathers will gladly involve themselves in the daily chores of infant rearing—feeding, bathing, changing diapers, and all the rest. And why not? There is nothing magical about handling a new baby. Nowhere has it been officially decreed that these tasks belong exclusively to a mother. The only exception I know of is breast-feeding, and in this case, the father can certainly be useful in taking care of the supplemental bottle feedings.

But I am afraid that too many fathers have been conditioned otherwise. A couple of weeks ago a new set of parents brought their baby into my office for his first monthly checkup. When I got to the examining room, mother and baby were waiting, but father was nowhere to be found. It turned out that the father was sitting by himself in the waiting room looking worried and nervous. After inviting him into the examining room, I asked why he had not come in with his family in the first place. He answered, "I was anxious to but I felt that I would be in the way." I pointed out that it was ridiculous for him to ever feel "in the way." I explained to him that it is important that he actively involve himself in all aspects of his baby's experiences and that this would help develop a happy, self-reliant child. As this family left my office, I was pleased to see that Poppa was proudly carrying his baby out the door.

THE ROLE OF THE NEW FATHER

Another factor that influences the role the new father takes is that many among us have been brainwashed to believe that it is somehow not manly for a father to feed or bathe his baby or change his diapers. This is utter nonsense. My own feelings are that just the opposite is true. I believe that it is not manly for a father to abdicate his role and just stand aside and watch. There is nothing unmasculine about loving and caring for your very own baby.

Raising a baby can best be accomplished as a cooperative venture in which both parents actively participate. I do not see this happening often enough, and it makes me both sad and angry. Obviously, sensible limits need to be set. For example, if a father comes home from work exhausted late at night and has to be up for an early morning appointment, he should not be expected to take care of the next 2 A.M. feeding. However, the important thing to strive for is active day-to-day involvement of both mother and father.

There is another very real advantage when the father is involved. With an experienced and competent father around to take care of his baby, a mother can leave when she wants to and remain in touch with the outside world. It is amazing that so many new mothers spend month after month staying home with their new babies without ever getting out. They lose contact with their friends and as a result feel deprived of all their other interests and activities.

It is really very simple. A father who is convinced that his involvement is necessary and wanted becomes active and cooperative. The benefits gained from such an attitude are enormous for the baby, for the mother, and for the marriage, as well as for the father.

I am happy to see that there has recently been a change in the attitude of more and more new fathers. This expanding group realizes how important it is for them to become involved in the day-to-day child-rearing experience. They anticipate with pleasure the opportunity to do their fair share of the work. And in doing so, they experience a great deal of pleasure and satisfaction. But I still find too many fathers who maintain a hands-off policy.

The real father figure is not the fellow who seldom touches his newborn baby, except when company arrives and he proudly lifts up the baby to show him off. The real father-figure is not the man who looks down on diaper changes, baths, and feedings as "woman's work." The real father figure is the man who, together with his wife, actively participates in taking care of his baby—working toward the goal of bringing up a healthy, happy, and self-reliant child. This is a difficult, full-time, but most fulfilling job. It requires total and equal participation from both parents. Pride in accomplishing it must be earned together and shared together.

SHOULD A MOTHER GO BACK TO WORK?

Many new mothers ask me whether or not they should go back to work. My answer to them is that it all depends on the particular needs and circumstances of each family. The question cannot be answered with a simple yes or no. It is a very important decision and requires careful thought and consideration.

There are three main reasons why new mothers choose to go back to work rather than to stay home and take care of their babies—economic demands, their own preference, and outside pressures.

1) **Economic demands:** With today's inflation, recession, and unemployment, many families just cannot make ends meet. Everybody wants the best for their children, but without sufficient funds this is virtually impossible to achieve. These are hard facts of life that many must face. In such cases I think the answer to whether or not Mother should go to work is obvious. She must go back to work. There is no choice. The problem that must be solved the best way possible is to find the

right parent substitute to properly care for the baby during the mother's working hours.

When Mr. and Mrs. T had their first baby, the father was still a full-time college student and only had a part-time job. Mrs. T worked full-time until two weeks before delivering her baby girl. She obviously had to resume working to support the needs of her now enlarged family. It all worked out beautifully—because Grandma T lived upstairs. Grandmothers can be ideal parent substitutes if they are physically well enough and properly motivated to do the job. One obvious advantage is that they don't receive any salary. This certainly was the case with Grandmother T. After one year, Mr. T finished college and found a good job. Mrs. T promptly quit her secretarial job and is now home with her baby, and loving every minute of it.

Opinion polls have shown that economics is the major determining factor as to why mothers go back to work. More than half the women who work would prefer to stay home. But the economics of life today forces them out of the house and back into the job market. No one ever need feel guilty about facing these hard realities.

2) **Preference:** Many mothers simply prefer to pursue a career outside the home rather than to make a career as a homemaker. I find this reasonable, and, if this is the case, I do not object. As a pediatrician, I am concerned with the health and well-being of children. It is obvious to me that a baby's health and well-being depends in large part on the parents' being happy and fulfilled. It makes no sense to force a new mother to remain home by instilling guilt, rather than allowing her to "do her thing." Guilt feelings just lead to a discontented, anxious, depressed mother who cannot, despite the best of intentions, give enough of herself to satisfy her baby's needs. Again, what is important in situations such as this is for the parents to carefully, without rushing, find the best possible parent substitute, so that the mother can go back to work with a clear conscience. Sometimes this

turns out to be Grandma, sometimes a housekeeper, sometimes a neighbor, sometimes a day-care center.

A new mother with a healthy four-month-old boy came in for the regular monthly checkup. The baby was thriving but despite this, it was clear that Mrs. S was disturbed and very uptight. I asked what was bothering her. She started to cry, and, after composing herself a bit, she told me that she was very anxious to go back to work. She had had a successful career as a buyer in a large department store, and she enjoyed her job and found it both fulfilling and interesting. But she was full of guilt about leaving her new baby. The problem was further complicated by the fact that so far she could not find a reliable person to care for her infant during the day. This case was an easy one for me to handle. I told her that unless and until the proper parent surrogate could be found, I would strongly advise her not to go back to work. When that reliable person was finally located, I would just as strongly recommend that she resume her career outside the house. Mrs. S would be unhappy and frustrated staying home, and she probably could not be the kind of mother her baby needed, no matter how hard she tried. It was clear that the entire family would be better off if Mrs. S went back to work. I tried to convince her not to feel guilty about her feelings—she has lots of company.

3) **Outside pressures:** In this day and age of the women's movement, women are being bombarded from all sides to emancipate themselves from the yoke of staying home to cook and clean. It is a most disturbing trend. New mothers are actually being made to feel guilty if they choose to remain home and try to be the best possible kind of mother for their children. I don't think I'm old-fashioned in believing that a baby is best off with a mother who stays home and who takes pride and satisfaction in the accomplishment of raising a healthy, happy baby. As far as I am concerned, there can be no more important or rewarding job. I get very upset when a new mother comes to see me looking a little sheepish and

tells me that she is going back to work, not because of the economics of her situation or because it is what she really prefers, but because she has been brainwashed into believing that in our present-day society returning to work is what is expected of any intelligent woman. This is complete nonsense. Some of the brightest and happiest women I know stay home and have a great time raising their children.

How many mothers actually do go back to work? The statistics are very interesting. In the United States, 38 percent of the total labor force of 91 million are female. Forty-one percent of the 64 million children under eighteen years of age have working mothers. Thirty-one percent of the 6 million children under six years of age have working mothers. So you can see that being a working mother is a real fact of life.

What do we know about what happens to the children of working mothers? In my experience and the experience of others, children of working mothers do just as well as those of nonworking mothers. As I have tried to explain, this is a complicated matter, and no two cases are alike. But if the proper parent surrogate is found, babies of working mothers grow up just as sound emotionally as do those of mothers who do not work.

I am firmly convinced that what babies and children need is *quality* care. The actual number of hours one spends with the child is not important. What is important is how the time is spent. A working mother who comes home contented and fulfilled after a good day's work and who then spends one hour with her baby in a happy, giving frame of mind, does more for her baby than the harrassed, dissatisfied mother who is home all day long with her baby, but wishes she were elsewhere.

What about guilt? In talking to many working mothers, what comes through most consistently is that most have some feelings of guilt about leaving their babies. I think that feeling guilty is wrong. There is no reason in the world for a mother to feel like that if she has chosen, for good reason, to go back to work. Deep down, most mothers feel that only they can give their babies the best possible loving care. I spend a good deal of my time trying to convince the working mother that there is no reason why they should feel guilt. Their babies will not grow up with psychological and emotional scars because they have chosen to work. A working mother is no less a mother because she spends a number of hours each day outside the house.

A common problem a working mother has to face, however, is old-fashioned fatigue. Having a full-time job outside the home as well as another almost full-time job at home can be physically very wearing. Many working mothers find themselves in a constant state of exhaustion. I think that some husbands are to blame for this. If a wife works, a father must assume his fair share of the work around the house. As I have mentioned, there is nothing unmanly about changing a baby's diapers or giving baby a bath. More and more young fathers are pitching in and working together with their wives in raising their babies. Fewer new fathers now come home after a day's work, sit down in front of the TV set with a bottle of beer, and wait for dinner to be served.

What about a father's preferences as to whether or not he wants his wife going back to work? It is all well and good for mothers to try to satisfy their own needs, whatever they may be. However, we should not lose sight of the fact that we are dealing with a family—a mother, a father, and a child. Some men feel very strongly about their wives working. A lot of extra tension is created in such cases. I think it is important that a mother and father communicate with each other to help arrive at a mutually satisfactory solution. In recent years, large inroads have been made in overcoming fathers' dissatisfaction with wives' going back to work. Fewer husbands take it as a personal affront when their wives decide that they would be happier working. Because this working mother trend is so widespread nowadays, it has become easier to accept, even by the most old-fashioned father. Fortunately, fewer fathers are shouting lately, "My wife will go back to work over my dead body."

Another question mothers frequently ask is how old should my baby be before I go back to work? There is no specific age. I have a female pediatrician friend who went back to work when each of her babies was two weeks old. I have to admit that her action is a little extreme, but it illustrates my position. There is no magic age that is best or worst for the baby. All the factors I have been discussing should be considered in arriving at a decision.

Every infant and child is entitled to receive loving and enthusiastic individual care. The fact that a mother works need not interfere with this. On the other hand, a woman should not be made to feel that she is a "social parasite" if she chooses to remain at home with her baby. Dr. Spock decries the ignominious standing given the job of child rearing in the United States. I agree with him wholeheartedly. The so-called career woman who looks down her nose at the mother who chooses to stay home with her baby has a lot to learn about life. Except for pressing economic reasons, a new mother should have a free choice in deciding what would be best for herself, her husband, and her baby. If the decision is made honestly and without outside pressures, it will turn out just fine for everybody. What you should aim for is a relaxed, happy, loving household. Whatever route you choose to help achieve that goal is the right one.

Common Problems and What to Do about Them

DIAPER RASH

Let me begin by telling you that almost all babies will develop some sort of diaper rash from time to time during the first few months of life. These rashes occur despite the most careful and conscientious care. Do not feel guilty if your baby becomes rashy—it probably is not your fault. I remember a new mother calling me one morning, practically hysterical. "Dr. Eden, what am I doing wrong? My baby has an awful diaper rash. I must be a terrible mother." Diaper rash is not a serious problem for the baby and should not cause you any concern. I will outline some simple suggestions for the prevention and treatment of these rashes a little later on in our discussion.

Diaper rashes have been with us for a very long time, and it is safe to assume that they will continue to remain with us (unless we figure out a way to toilet-train our babies before leaving the hospital nursery). In reviewing what has been written about diaper rash in the medical literature, the first reference I could find dates back to 1877, so for about one hundred years (and no doubt for much longer than that) babies wearing diapers have developed red bottoms and fronts. All these rashes cleared up eventually.

Why do so many babies wearing diapers become rashy? First of all, the baby's skin is very sensitive and, therefore, very susceptible to rashes; so diaper rash is often unavoidable. Add to this the fact that the skin beneath the diaper is almost continuously wet from urine and from stool. It is indeed surprising that there are times when the baby is free of rash.

No matter how excellent the skin care of the newborn baby may be, a certain number of babies will become rashy. Many new mothers bring their babies home from the hospital with a full-blown diaper rash and are very upset about this. Please do not blame the hospital nurse—it is usually unavoidable.

By far the most common cause of diaper rash is the constant wetness of the baby's tender, sensitive skin. The wet diaper causes irritation, and this shortly leads to the skin's becoming red and rough. This continuous contact of the skin with the moist diaper results in water-logging of the skin and finally the rash. With this in mind, treatment becomes fairly obvious. Simply change your baby's diaper more frequently, that is, as soon as it feels slightly damp. The irritated area should be thoroughly cleansed and exposed to the air. During the day, this is best achieved when the baby is napping. Place a folded diaper under him and allow the warm air to dry the bare skin of the diaper area. It can also be helpful to use a soothing ointment or cream over the affected area. In most cases you will be pleasantly surprised by how rapidly the rash clears up.

A word of caution about cleaning the diaper area. It is important not to scrub the sensitive skin too vigorously, since this will only cause additional irritation and lead to a more severe rash. I can illustrate this point with a recent experience in my office.

A new mother came with tears in her eyes, terribly

worried and disturbed. Her two-month-old baby had a diaper rash that kept getting worse despite the fact that she had been following my instructions explicitly for two weeks. After questioning her carefully, the reason for the trouble became clear. It turned out that Mamma was trying too hard. She was changing her baby's diaper every thirty minutes whether it was wet or dry, and each time she vigorously scrubbed down the affected area. As a result, the skin became more irritated and red. Gentle handling is the key to successful treatment!

The second main cause of diaper rash is ammonia formation beneath the diaper. This usually develops after the baby is six months old. The ammonia is produced from the urine by the action on it by a certain normal bacteria found in the feces called "bacillus ammoniagenes." Most mothers have no trouble in making the diagnosis of ammonia diaper rash. When changing baby's diaper, there is a strong ammonia smell, often so strong as to cause actual tearing of the eyes. This, plus noticing a rash, makes the diagnosis clear. The warm, wet diapers are an excellent environment for the growth of this bacteria; so more and more ammonia is produced, and the ammonia acts as an irritant to the skin and produces a rash.

Your physician should be consulted as to what specific steps should be taken to get rid of the ammonia. It may be necessary to wash out your diapers with an antiseptic to kill off the bacteria, or specially treated diapers may be used. The use of disposable diapers can also be effective. Again, the main standby of treatment is frequent diaper changes and exposure to air.

There are two additional main causes of diaper rash.

1) Loose bowel movements which irritate the skin around the anus and buttocks. Most important is to determine the cause of the diarrhea and to treat it accordingly. Your physician must be consulted. As soon as the bowel movements become normal in consistency, the rash disappears.

2) Low water intake. When a baby drinks little or no water, his urine may become too concentrated and acidy, and this can cause skin irritation and rash. It all clears up speedily by giving the baby extra water feedings.

A frequently asked question about diaper rash is related to cloth versus disposable diapers. Is one type of diaper superior to the other? I have no real preference. By and large, babies do just as well with either type. When a diaper rash does develop, the use of any rubber or plastic covering should be eliminated. These tend to retain liquid and prevent evaporation and do not allow air to reach the irritated skin.

In the treatment of diaper rash, the following steps should be taken:

1) Change diapers frequently, as soon as they are damp.

2) Gently and thoroughly clean the involved area.

3) Expose the rashy skin to the air as often and for as long as possible.

4) Remove any rubber or plastic diaper covering during the day.

5) If a strong ammonia smell is present, treat the diapers with an antiseptic or use disposable diapers.

6) Give your baby extra water.

7) If the rash is severe or if it persists, consult your physician.

Diaper rash should be kept in proper perspective. In almost all cases, it is not serious and should not cause any worry. It cannot hurt your baby and usually does not cause your baby any pain, and it will clear up with proper care. Most times it does not require bringing your baby to your doctor—his telephone advice is sufficient. If, however, the rash spreads or becomes worse (for example, if the skin becomes fiery red or looks raw and wet), then it is necessary for your physician to examine the baby. Based on the character and distribution of the rash, he can then prescribe specific treatment.

Almost all babies will develop a diaper rash sooner or later, and they always clear up; so my best advice is to relax and enjoy your baby—red bottom and all.

COLIC

Colic simply means recurrent pain in the abdomen or bowels. In order to understand the problem and how to cope with it, let me first give you a brief description of how a baby with colic acts.

A baby who has previously been peaceful and contented will suddenly start to cry loudly and continually and will pull up or stiffen her legs. She will also usually have a distended or swollen abdomen due to gas. The crying and screaming continues without letup and may last for hours. Then it finally stops just as suddenly as it started. These colic attacks usually occur in the evening or during the night, and after they are over, the baby is again perfectly fine until the next episode which begins the following evening, often at exactly the same time. I once received a late night telephone call from the mother of a two-month-old. "I'm sorry to wake you at such an ungodly hour, but I don't know what to do with my colicky baby." Half asleep, I asked her what time it was. She answered, "My watch is broken, but I know it's 1:30

A.M." Well, my watch was working fine, and indeed it was 1:30 A.M.

I am not describing the so-called fussy baby who frets, cries a little, whimpers, and takes a long time to settle down and go to sleep. I am talking about prolonged, loud crying spells during which it is obvious that the baby is in pain. These episodes repeat themselves over and over again. The usual story of colic is a baby who has had no long crying periods in the nursery or during the first few days at home. When she is one or two weeks old, the colic begins and continues steadily almost every day. Happily, it is all over in the great majority of cases by the time the baby reaches three months of age. Thus, it is often called "three-month colic."

There are many theories as to what causes colic, but so far they are only theories—we just don't know why it happens, and why some babies are affected and others are not. It may be associated with hunger or with swallowed air which has passed into the intestine. Overfeeding may cause distention and discomfort. Since most of the attacks occur in the evening, fatigue may play a part.

Certainly, there is no one factor which consistently causes colic. What is clear from my experience is that an overly tense, worried, or angry household more often produces a colicky baby than does a relaxed and peaceful environment. However, this does not always hold true. Recently, one of my calmest, sweetest mothers had her third baby, who turned out to have severe colic.

It is most important for mothers to understand that colic is not a disease or illness, and it will not hurt your baby in any way! Long periods of nonstop loud crying cannot hurt your baby, but it will finally tire her out enough so that she will fall asleep. As I often tell my distraught mothers, crying is good exercise and perfectly normal in colic. I also remind my mothers that the colic will almost always be over by the time the baby is three months old.

These babies grow and develop normally and literally

thrive during this most trying period. Mamma is usually the one exhausted by it all. As a matter of fact, when the colic is finally over, these babies become model citizens—contented, alert, and loveable. Colic babies are healthy, bright babies with excellent appetites, and their parents should remember this during this difficult two- to three-month period.

Once your physician has diagnosed colic in your baby, what can be done about it? In discussing this subject with many of my pediatrician friends, it turns out that each of us has his favorite remedies. Here are some effective methods.

1) Put your baby on her stomach across your lap on a heating pad or hot water bottle. Sometimes just rubbing your baby's abdomen will help.

2) Help your baby expel or pass gas, either by gently inserting an infant suppository or lubricated thermometer tip into the rectum.

3) Play music or run your vacuum cleaner. Why this often helps I do not know, but it certainly can be effective in some cases.

4) Give your baby fennel seed tea. If there is a grandmother in the house, she will know about this time-honored remedy for relieving the gassy baby. Simply bring one pint of water to a boil, pour over one teaspoon fennel tea, cool, strain, and give to baby.

5) Use a pacifier. Some babies continue to scream despite the above methods and only calm down by means of a pacifier. With such a baby, this is a good treatment.

6) Give a mild sedative. A certain number of babies with colic cannot be helped except by using specific medication. Your physician will decide if medicine is necessary and, if so, will prescribe the proper dose of a mild sedative which will be perfectly safe for your baby.

Many mothers believe that changing the baby's formula will solve the problem. In my experience this is not the case. The fact is that colic occurs in breast-fed babies and in bottle-fed babies on all sorts of different formulas. It is clear that the type of milk the baby takes is not the cause of colic. If it were, why should the baby take all her other milk feedings without trouble and start her painful crying only with the evening bottle? If the milk were the cause, each feeding during the day would give her trouble.

Of course, your physician must be the one to make the diagnosis of colic, since there are many other causes of prolonged crying to be considered. But once you are told that your baby has colic, it is most important to adjust to the situation. It is very difficult for a mother to listen to her baby cry for long periods of time. Nevertheless, you must realize that crying is normal in colic and cannot hurt your baby in any way. Knowing that it will be over by the time your baby is three months old makes it easier to cope with the problem.

A final word of advice: With the knowledge that colic is not a disease and, therefore, nothing to worry about, relax and stop worrying. A baby with colic is healthy. Once you accept this, you will be amazed by how much the whole situation will be improved.

VOMITING

One of the most poorly understood subjects facing new parents is the problem of vomiting. This is especially true during the first few months of life. Many parents have no idea what vomiting actually means and what should be done about it. Through the years it has become more and more obvious to me that this is one area that requires much clarification. Too many parents cannot differentiate between vomiting, "spitting up," and "cheesing." This causes a lot of extra worrying for no good reason. The best way to start our discussion is to define some terms.

1) **Vomiting:** By this I mean the ejection of large amounts of the stomach contents through the mouth. Doctors often use the term "projectile vomiting" to describe the forceful regurgitation of the vomitus. Such a condition requires medical evaluation. Persistent vomiting must not be ignored.

2) **Spitting up:** This condition describes the gentle

"spilling out" of small amounts of stomach contents shortly after a feeding. It is very common during the first few months of life and is considered completely normal and so does not require treatment.

3) **Cheesing:** This refers to the "spitting up" of curdled milk. If milk remains in the stomach for any length of time, it becomes acidified by the acids normally found in the stomach, and this process causes the milk to curdle. Therefore, the "cheesing" occurs about one hour after a feeding and is frequently seen in babies who are poor burpers. Again, this is normal and does not need to be treated in any way.

Just about every infant will spit up or cheese at one time or another, and some babies do much more than others. Neither condition interferes in any way with the baby's normal growth and development. Teething often causes the baby to spit up or cheese more than usual because of the swallowing of excessive amounts of saliva. Both conditions are self-limiting and stop by themselves, usually by the time the baby is sitting up (six to eight months of age). It is, therefore, important that you be able to differentiate between spitting up, cheesing, and real vomiting. Persistent vomiting requires consultation with your baby's physician, while spitting up and cheesing usually do not.

I'd like to answer some questions that mothers ask me frequently.

What are the usual causes of spitting up during the first few months of a baby's life?

1) Overfeeding: This is probably the most common cause of spitting up. Simply giving the baby too much milk overloads the stomach and results in the baby "spilling out" some of the extra fluid.

2) Underburping: Some babies just don't burp as easily or readily as others, and this also can result in spitting up shortly after a feeding.

3) **Poor positioning:** If the baby is not held properly during the feeding or is put down too soon after the feeding, spitting up can result.

4) **Feeding too rapidly:** If you allow your baby to swallow too much air during her feeding, she has a tendency to spit up. You must remember that there is no air in the bottle—the baby takes in air around the nipple (bottle or breast).

5) **Sudden jostling or squeezing:** If your baby is not handled gently enough, spitting up may take place.

6) **A nervous mother:** It has been my experience that mothers who are tense and nervous while feeding their babies often have "spitters."

7) **The digestive motions of the stomach:** In some cases normal digestive motions within the baby's stomach can result in spitting up.

What are the usual causes of cheesing during the first few months?

As I have stated, milk curdles when it is acted upon by the acids normally found in the stomach. If the baby regurgitates about an hour following the feeding, curdled milk is what comes up. Often babies who are poor burpers have a tendency to do a lot of cheesing, and if this happens often enough, it gives the house a characteristic odor of a cheese factory. No one really understands why some babies do a lot of cheesing and others do not. This is not a medical problem. You simply have the nuisance of having to change sheets and shirts frequently and of figuring out how to get rid of the odor in the house.

What are some of the important causes of real vomiting during the first few months of life?

1) **Infection:** An infection anywhere in the body can cause vomiting. Often the infection is in the gastrointestinal tract (for example, intestinal flu), but the infection does not always have to be in the gut. For example, it is quite characteristic for a baby with an ear infection to do a lot of vomiting.

2) **Milk allergy:** A small percentage of infants are actually allergic to the cow's milk protein. This allergy can manifest itself by persistent vomiting. If, in fact, the cause of the vomiting is allergy, then switching the baby to a milk substitute, such as one of the soybean or meat base preparations, will clear up the situation. Of course, your physician is the one to determine whether or not milk allergy is the cause of the trouble.

3) **Intestinal obstruction:** Fortunately, this rarely occurs, but when it does, it is a real emergency. There are many causes of obstruction, and immediate hospitalization with appropriate laboratory and X-ray procedures is essential. The baby who has intestinal obstruction vomits persistently, occasionally with bile (green in color) in the vomitus. The abdomen is often swollen or distended, and there is pained crying and screaming.

Obviously, there are many, many other causes of vomiting, but for our purposes it is not necessary to list them all.

What should be done if your baby is vomiting a great deal?

1) Take the baby's temperature.
2) Examine the character of the material vomited. Look especially for greenish material (bile) and for blood.
3) Look at the baby's abdomen to see whether or not it is swollen.
4) Examine the groin area for any lumps or masses. If present, they may represent an inguinal hernia.
5) Call your physician and report your findings.

A sudden change in the amount of regurgitation should alert you to the possibility of trouble. For example, if a baby who previously was only spitting up small amounts suddenly starts to vomit the entire contents of each feeding forcefully, you must report this to your doctor without delay.

When should your doctor be called?

When there is

1) Projectile vomiting
2) Persistent vomiting (especially if the baby's diapers remain dry)
3) Bile or blood in the vomitus
4) Vomiting associated with pain
5) Vomiting associated with a swollen abdomen
6) Vomiting associated with sudden appearance of a lump or mass in the groin
7) Vomiting associated with fever
8) Vomiting associated with diarrhea

All the above are real danger signals and require your immediate recognition and medical consultation. If you have any question in your mind about the vomiting, it is safest to call your baby's doctor.

What about treatment?

In the case of spitting up and/or cheesing, there is really nothing that need be done. These infants gain at the normal rate, and aside from using extra linen, diapers, and air fresheners, there is nothing else to do. When real vomiting occurs, however, the cause of the vomiting must be found so that appropriate treatment can be given; your doctor must be notified. If the vomiting is associated with a gastrointestinal infection (and a good clue to this would be associated diarrhea and fever), giving the baby small sips of clear fluid (water or tea) often settles the stomach and stops the vomiting. Your physician may prescribe specific medication for this purpose, which at times is given by mouth and other times via suppository.

I'd like to tell you about a recent case that I think illustrates the confusion. A new mother with a five-month-old baby called me one Sunday morning, frantic with worry. "Dr. Eden, my baby vomits everything he eats. Nothing stays down. This has been going on for days. What should I do?" I met her and the baby in my office one hour later. The baby had gained 2 1/2 pounds since the last visit three weeks before. The baby looked fine except that he was somewhat overweight. The physical examination was completely within normal limits. With further discussion, I found out that the baby was having six or seven normal bowel movements each day and was taking in enormous quantities of milk and solid food. The "vomiting" that the mother was so worried about was not vomiting at all; it simply was a persistent spitting up after every feeding, obviously due to overfeeding. Every time the baby spit up, mama immediately re-fed him. This, of course, caused more spitting up. It took me quite a while to convince this mother that her baby would not starve before the next feeding despite the spitting up.

Almost all babies do some spitting up or cheesing, and the sooner new parents realize this, the better for all concerned—the baby, the parents, and the doctor.

CONSTIPATION

There is only one sensible way to approach this topic. This is to discuss briefly the usual patterns of stool evacuation during a baby's first few months of life. Only by understanding what is considered normal will you be able to decide when and if your baby is actually constipated. Many new parents have very strange ideas about this subject. By the end of this chapter, I hope you will have a better understanding of constipation and, if your baby does develop it, be competent to recognize and treat it.

Too many new mothers are overly concerned, and at times actually obsessed, with bowel movements of their babies. It almost seems as if their every waking moment is taken up with a careful examination and analysis of each dirty diaper. Many well-meaning parents even keep carefully written records—number, color, odor, consistency, etc. This compulsion is unnecessary—a complete waste of time and effort. The result is undue worry and tension for everybody. Obviously, I am not talking about a situation when your physician has specifically asked that you keep such a diary. But you don't need to take it upon yourself to be superefficient BM scorekeeper.

Let me give you an example that will illustrate what I mean by fecal overfixation. I hold a telephone advice session each day. During this specified morning hour, my patients call me directly with questions and problems. Just for the fun of it, I kept a record of the topics brought up each day for a week. The number of daily phone calls ranged between twenty and twenty-five. Would you believe that close to one-half of all the calls related to stools? Incidentally, of all the bowel-movement-related "problems" of that week, only two required my seeing the baby. The misconceptions that parents have continue to surprise and amaze me. So let us begin to learn what is normal and what you may expect from your new baby.

There is no such thing as an average daily number of stools for a baby. Each baby has her own average. Some may have up to twelve normal bowel movements each day. Other babies may average one normal stool every three days. If you took one hundred babies and averaged their stools per day, you would come up with a figure of three to four, but this number is meaningless as far as your own one baby is concerned. And the specific number of normal bowel movements per day is in no way related to the health or well-being of the baby.

As a rule, the breast-fed baby has more frequent stools than the one who is bottle-fed. Many babies have a bowel movement after each feeding, but just as many do not. Just remember that the number of stools per day is of absolutely no importance.

During the baby's first few months of life, her stools are usually soft and unformed (salvelike in consistency) and often leave a water ring around the diaper. The bottle-fed baby often has a somewhat firmer stool than that of the baby who is breast-fed. The breast-fed infant's stool is usually pale yellow to light brown.

Occasionally, the stools may be greenish in color, but this is no cause for alarm. There are a couple of explanations for the green stool. When food passes through the infant's intestine too rapidly, the bile (green in color), which is secreted from the liver into the intestine, does not have enough time to be changed in color to yellow or brown by the digestive process. Another reason for the green stool is the fact that an infant's bile is normally secreted in spurts rather than at a regular rate, so if a large squirt of bile happens to pass into the gut, it will color that particular stool green. However, if your baby always has green stools, this should be reported to your doctor.

The best definition of constipation I can give you comes straight out of my medical dictionary: "The difficult evacuation or the retention of feces." If your baby has unusually firm, marblelike stools, she is constipated. If her stools become more infrequent and harder than usual, she is constipated. When your baby is in obvious pain during the passage of a rocklike bowel movement, she is constipated. When this difficulty in the passage of the feces is accompanied by a bloated or distended abdomen, your physician must be called immediately. The key to recognizing constipation is a change from your baby's usual number and consistency to fewer and harder stools.

Most new babies do some grunting and straining during stool evacuation, and they often turn quite red from their efforts. These antics are considered normal and are not signs of constipation, provided the bowel movement itself is soft.

Infants have very small, tight anal openings, so some straining is to be expected. As a matter of fact, this is nature's way of gradually stretching the opening. Occasionally, the sphincter will just be too tight to allow the stool to pass through, and the straining may cause a small tear with resultant bloody streaks on the diaper or stool. This happens once in a while and is no cause for panic. Simply coat the area with a liberal quantity of petroleum jelly or a bland ointment and notify your doctor. He may have to stretch the opening manually. This can be done in his office and takes just a couple of minutes.

If your baby is truly constipated during the period of 100 percent milk feedings (bottle or breast), simply add a little sugar to the water she drinks. One-half teaspoon of sugar to two ounces of water is quite effective. If your baby remains constipated, the time has come to discuss it with your physician so that he may determine the specific cause. If your baby has been constipated from the time she was brought home from the hospital, this also necessitates your doctor's involvement. In my experience, breast-fed babies are seldom constipated. When the baby is switched from breast or formula to whole milk, stools usually become firmer, and actual constipation may result.

When solid foods are added to the diet, a number of babies suddenly become constipated. In these cases I would suggest using prune juice—one ounce mixed with one ounce water. Alternative methods would be giving prune pulp, apricots, or bran-containing cereals. While your baby is constipated, eliminate rice or barley cereal and bananas, all of which have a tendency to be binding. Some pediatricians advocate a very mild artificial laxative such as one teaspoon of milk of magnesia. I personally prefer the use of the natural laxatives contained in the foods mentioned above.

There may be times when a glycerine suppository or enema may be necessary. These methods should be carried out only after consultation with your doctor.

It is not uncommon for a baby to become constipated when she is ill. Fever itself predisposes a baby to constipation. When a baby is sick, she eats less, and this also can lead to her becoming constipated.

There are situations related to constipation about which your doctor should be called. These are (1) any sudden change in the usual stool pattern; (2) continuous constipation since birth; (3) actual pain while trying to have a bowel movement, especially if her abdomen is distended; (4) bloody or black bowel movements.

There is no law that states that your baby must produce a certain specific number of bowel movements a day. The "regularity" phobia—the "one bowel movement per day or you are in trouble" concept—is absolute nonsense for infants and children (as well as for adults). There is no reason to carefully examine each and every soiled diaper. I can think of a lot more pleasant and meaningful ways to spend one's time. Try looking at your baby's face for a change. Stop counting bowel movements! Learn what is normal for your baby, and learn what foods are best for maintaining her normal evacuation pattern. That's all there is to it.

After finishing this chapter, I received the following 11 P.M. telephone call from a frantic mother. It summed up perfectly what I've been trying to get across to you. "Dr. Eden, I am scared out of my wits. Michael, my eight-week-old, had seven rather than his usual six bowel movements today." I asked how she could be so sure about the exact number. She answered: "Not only am I sure, I'm 100 percent positive. Don't you realize that I have kept track of every single bowel movement my baby has had since I brought him home from the hospital?"

DIARRHEA

The words "diarrhea" and "dehydration" are terrifying to many parents of infants and young babies. I'd like to eliminate this fear by explaining some simple facts and concepts about this subject. This information will also help you to manage the problem if and when it develops.

I would like to start off by making a general observation. In my experience, too many mothers spend too much of their time carefully examining, counting, smelling, and describing their infants' bowel movements. During an English course I took while in college, we had a discussion about the usage of words in various languages. The point was made that the value systems of the culture determine the frequency of the particular word usage. Our professor pointed out that in the United States the single word that has the most synonyms, colloquialisms, and slang expressions describing it was "money." On the other hand, Eskimo language has the greatest number of different words to describe snow. As far as I am concerned, money may be Number One in the United

States, but bowel movements run a close second. Our culture has some strange value systems indeed. What I am trying to say is that more time should be spent watching how your baby acts, and less time should be devoted to the careful scrutiny of each and every one of your infant's stools.

Hippocrates, the famous Greek physician who is considered the father of medicine, born in the year 460 B.C., wrote: "Diarrhea is the abnormal liquidity and frequency of fecal discharges." Nobody has yet come up with a better definition.

Diarrhea means that the stools are looser, more watery, and more frequent than normal. It follows that the key to recognizing true diarrhea is knowing what is *normal* for your baby. A change from this normal pattern to more watery and more frequent BMs equals diarrhea.

A common misconception is believing that a baby having more than four or five stools a day has diarrhea. This is nonsense. Many babies have an evacuation after each feeding, and this is perfectly normal. Other infants have one BM every three days, and this also is normal. I remember two consecutive phone calls during one of my telephone advice hours. Mother Number One reported that her baby usually had eight BMs daily but that they were normal in consistency. Mother Number Two told me that her baby had three green, watery, explosive stools during the previous night. Obviously, the baby with the three BMs had diarrhea, and the baby with eight stools did not. Learn your baby's normal stool pattern. If it changes, you will be alert to the possibility of the beginning of diarrhea. But this change must be significant.

Let me give you an example that illustrates what I mean by a significant change. At five minutes past midnight my phone rang. Mrs. G reported that baby John had passed seven BMs the previous day instead of his usual six. After determining that the baby was acting fine and that the stools were in fact normal in consistency, I asked her the sixty-four-thousand-dollar question: "How is it you called me at 12:05 A.M.?" Her answer: "Dr. Eden, you know very well that each day ends at midnight, and so my daily BM diary ends at midnight."

Let's start at the beginning. The newborn first passes meconium. This is a dark, thick, black-green substance that is normally excreted during the first couple of days of life. Then comes the period of transitional stools—loose, yellow-green, and full of mucus. This type of stool continues for the next three or four days. By around seven days of age the new baby begins to pass the typical "milk" stool. Since many newborns are discharged from hospital nurseries at three or four days of age, they come home during the transitional stool period. I have received many frantic phone calls from mothers who have just not been aware that this is normal and is not diarrhea.

Breast-fed babies have softer, less firm stools than those of bottle-fed infants. Both breast- and bottle-fed babies have softer, less formed stools than older children and adults, and usually these stools are characterized by a diaper water ring around them.

Here are the most common causes of infant diarrhea:

1) **Overfeeding:** In my experience, this is the number one cause of mild diarrhea during the first few months. It must always be kept in mind when your baby's stools become looser or more frequent than usual. Incidentally, overfeeding can also lead to vomiting. All that you need to do is reduce the intake, and the diarrhea will quickly subside.

2) **Teething:** Many babies have a pattern of mild diarrhea with every new tooth. Many times mothers can actually predict when the next tooth is coming through by this change in the normal BM pattern. The explanation for this that makes the most sense is that a large amount of saliva is manufactured during teething. Much of it is swallowed and, therefore, dilutes the stool and makes it looser.

3) **Food intolerance:** Some infants are unable to tolerate cow's milk or some specific solid food. The body's reaction to this food allergy may be to develop diarrhea. If you remove the offending milk or food from the diet, the diarrhea rapidly improves.

4) **Antibiotics:** Bacterial infections are treated with different antibiotics. One of their side effects is diarrhea. If this happens, it may be necessary to stop the medication or to switch to another antibiotic. Of course, your doctor is the one to make this decision for you.

5) **Parenteral disease:** This refers to any illness not related to the gastrointestinal tract, as, for example, the common cold (upper respiratory infection). Any of these can trigger off diarrhea. The diarrhea accompanying a parenteral disease is controlled as soon as the baby recovers from the illness. Incidentally, it is always a good idea to increase the fluid intake and decrease the solid foods when your baby is ill with fever. In such situations the fever causes increased water loss, and so more fluids by mouth are needed to compensate.

6) **Gastrointestinal infections:** Any viral or bacterial infection of the gastrointestinal tract obviously will cause diarrhea (and often vomiting as well). This form of diarrhea can be severe and often is associated with fever and with blood or mucus in the stool. In such cases, your doctor should immediately be called. He may prescribe specific medication, or he may want to see the baby.

7) **Unexplained:** There are a number of babies who develop periodic episodes of diarrhea for no apparent reason. This diarrhea is mild and always clears up by itself.

If your baby's stools are looser and more frequent than usual but he is acting well and taking his feedings normally without vomiting or fever, the chances are you are dealing with a case of mild diarrhea. Further evidence suggesting that the diarrhea is not severe would be good color, a lusty and vigorous cry, and a normal amount of urine. The great majority of cases of diarrhea in infancy fall into this category.

There are a number of different methods to treat diarrhea. The basic approach common to all is to reduce the number of calories you give the baby. Some physicians prefer the starvation method. This consists of withholding all solid food for a twelve- to twenty-four-hour period and giving only boiled water or weak tea during this time. The purpose is to decrease the peristaltic activity of the intestine as well as to decrease the volume of the stool. Unless the baby is also vomiting, I personally do not recommend this method. When the diarrhea is associated with vomiting, I omit one or two feedings, and this usually stops the vomiting. In treating diarrhea without vomiting, I prefer the feeding method—giving the baby milk or formula diluted with equal parts of water. The baby should not be fed too frequently. It has been shown that very frequent feedings, such as every hour or two, activates the gastro-colic reflex, and this leads to further diarrhea and more loss of water and salt. The diluted milk or formula should be sufficiently warmed, since ice cold fluids increase intestinal activity and aggravate the problem.

Some pediatricians suggest the use of one of the commercially available electrolyte solutions, and others use a sugar-water mixture. Still others prefer using skim milk. Since there are so many approaches to the management of diarrhea, I would suggest that you check with your own doctor and find out what method he recommends.

An infant or baby with diarrhea usually loses his appetite for solid food. You should never coax or force such a baby to eat. It is much more important that he be offered fluids. When solids are pushed too vigorously, they can cause vomiting, and that is the last thing you want to happen. But if your baby is hungry for solids, I would restrict the diet to mashed, ripe banana or scraped apple. Both of these foods have a high pectin content, which is helpful in reducing diarrhea. Rice cereal is also binding and may safely be given. Do not give medication to the baby on your own. Your physician will prescribe the appropriate drug if he feels it is needed to treat the diarrhea.

As the diarrhea improves, the diluted milk or formula should be gradually strengthened. After twenty-four hours of normal stools, I allow full-strength formula or milk to be restarted. After another twenty-four hours of normal BMs, I allow the regular prediarrhea solid-food diet to be reinstituted. It is a good idea to keep in touch with your physician via daily telephone progress reports.

If you even suspect that your infant or baby has more than a mild form of diarrhea, it is important that you notify your physician. He will be interested in knowing the following:

1) Age of baby
2) Stools—number, character, blood or mucus?
3) When did the diarrhea begin?
4) Vomiting?
5) Fever?
6) Normal or decreased amount of urine?
7) Taking fluids well or poorly?
8) Cranky and irritable or happy and contented?

Your answers will help your doctor decide how severe the problem is and what should be done about it.

Diarrhea becomes an emergency when your baby shows evidence of dehydration. Dehydration means the excessive loss of fluids from the body. This loss is primarily one of salt (sodium and chloride) and water. In addition, vital electrolytes (chemicals) in the blood are also affected. The result of this is a disruption of the delicate balance necessary to maintain normal bodily functions. If the dehydration becomes severe enough, it can cause the baby to go into shock. This must not be permitted to happen, since shock is life-threatening to the baby.

With severe diarrhea a great deal of water and salt is lost via the stools, and dehydration may result. If severe diarrhea is also associated with vomiting, the dehydration can develop even more rapidly, since fluids are being lost in two directions. Whatever the cause, dehydration can be extremely dangerous and requires prompt and vigorous treatment. Therefore, any significant degree of dehydration must be considered an emergency. In order to rapidly replace the lost water and electrolytes by intravenous solutions, hospitalization is required. Fortunately this method of treatment is very effective, and the dehydration can usually be rapidly corrected.

Infants and babies require more fluid per pound of body weight than do older children and adults in order to maintain their normal metabolism. Therefore, they are more susceptible to dehydration. Infants need 2 1/2 ounces of fluid per pound of weight each twenty-four hours. An older child needs about half as much fluid per pound of his weight, and an adult needs only one-fifth as much. For example, a ten-pound infant requires twenty-five ounces of fluid per day. If this infant takes in much less than this amount or if he loses a lot of his body fluids through watery bowel movements or from vomiting, he will fall behind his requirements much more rapidly than the older child or adult. What this means is that the younger the baby, the easier and quicker it is for dehydration to develop.

You must be able to recognize the signs and symptoms of dehydration. These are:

1) Change in behavior—listless and sleepy or very irritable
2) Decreased amount of urine
3) Fever
4) Depressed anterior fontanel (soft spot on top of the head)

5) Sunken eyeballs
6) Dry lips, tongue, and skin
7) Poor sucking
8) Gray color to skin
9) Rapid breathing and fast pulse
10) Weight loss

When and if your baby develops any of the above signs and symptoms along with his diarrhea, dehydration must be suspected. Call your physician immediately. While waiting for his return call, keep the baby cool and try to give him some clear fluids by mouth (water or tea). If your doctor is not available, the best advice I can give you is to take the baby to the nearest hospital emergency room for examination. It may turn out to be a false alarm, but, if your baby is truly dehydrated, he requires immediate treatment.

I would like to end this chapter by re-emphasizing the following points:

1) Learn your baby's normal stool pattern.
2) Most cases of infant diarrhea are mild and easily controlled.
3) If you suspect severe diarrhea, call your doctor.
4) Remember the signs and symptoms of dehydration.
5) The baby's general behavior is more important than the number of his stools.
6) If you must count, let it be your blessings!

TEMPERATURE

Parents are always asking me what I consider a baby's normal temperature. My answer is that there is no such thing as a specific normal temperature. There is a range of normal temperatures, which, incidentally, is the same for babies, children, and adults.

The whole topic of temperature and fever is confusing and frightening to many new parents. I have spent a great deal of time through the years discussing this subject with my patients. I'd like to share this experience with you. To best accomplish this, let me answer the following questions:

What is the difference between temperature and fever?

I'd like to have a quarter (it used to be a nickel before inflation) for every time I have heard "Dr. Eden, my baby has a temperature. What should I do?" Temperature refers to the degree of heat in our bodies, while fever means an elevated temperature above the normal range. All of us always have temperature, but we only occasionally have fever.

What is the normal range of temperature?

I would consider a rectal temperature of between 97°

and 100° to be within the normal range. If the thermometer reads over 100° (and your baby has been at rest for at least a half hour before the temperature taking), this usually indicates fever.

What about that 98.6° mark on the thermometer?

It is unfortunate that all thermometers have that magic arrow pointing to 98.6°. This arrow causes a good deal of undue concern and worry. The fact of the matter is that there is nothing special about 98.6°. Just remember the normal range and not a specific number. For example, a temperature of 99.4° is just as normal as a 98.6° reading. Anything below 100° is fine.

What kind of thermometer should I use?

A rectal thermometer, at least until your youngster is three years old. Taking the temperature orally can be risky if the child is too young. She can easily bite or break off the bulb. Further, an oral temperature is accurate only if the thermometer is kept under the tongue, and a child below age three will usually not cooperate. There are two types of thermometers, oral (mouth) and rectal. The only difference between them is the shape of the bulb at the top. The rectal thermometer has a round, smooth bulb, while the oral one has a long, slender bulb (see illustrations). The reason for the difference in shape is obvious—safety and efficiency. It is possible to use the two types of thermometers interchangeably, but I would strongly recommend that you don't do it. The oral thermometer can break off more easily in the rectum if the baby suddenly jumps or squirms. If the rectal thermometer is used in the mouth, you must, of course, first clean it off thoroughly with alcohol.

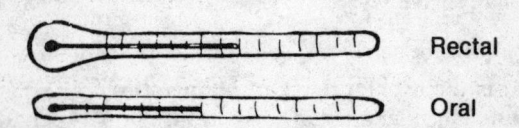

Rectal

Oral

Is there a difference between the rectal and the oral temperature readings?

Yes there is. The rectal temperature is usually about one degree higher. I might add that the axillary (underarm) temperature, which occasionally may be used, lies somewhere between the oral and rectal reading. A fairly accurate reading may be obtained by this method; place the bulb of either type of thermometer in the baby's armpit and hold that arm flat against her chest.

How long should a thermometer be kept in?

One minute is sufficient for a rectal temperature. In fact, you can get a pretty accurate reading after just fifteen to twenty seconds. I will never forget what happened to me one evening a couple of years ago. My wife and I were about to leave for the theatre when a worried mother called to report that she thought her nine-month-old was sick. The baby felt "warm," and she did not know what to do. I suggested that she take the baby's temperature and call me right back. Fifteen minutes elapsed and nothing happened. With the help of my telephone answering service, I tracked down her telephone number and called back. Why hadn't she called back? You guessed it. The thermometer was still in the baby's bottom and had been there for a full ten minutes. "I thought I should get an accurate reading, and so I left it in a bit longer than usual just to be on the safe side." You might be happy to know that the baby's temperature was 98° and that we managed to get to the theatre on time. Oral temperature readings require two minutes, while axillary temperatures take three to four minutes for accurate results.

How should a baby's temperature be taken?

1) Shake down the thermometer until the mercury column is below the arrow.

2) Put a little petroleum jelly on the bulb.

3) Place the baby on her stomach, preferably over

your knees—or on her side with her knees slightly drawn up.

4) Push the thermometer gently into the rectum about one inch.

5) Keep your palm flat over her buttocks holding the thermometer lightly between two fingers (as in holding a cigarette, before you stopped smoking).

6) After one minute, gently withdraw the thermometer and wipe it off with a tissue. Never clean off the thermometer in hot water.

7) After reading the temperature, shake down to below the arrow and clean with alcohol.

How do you read the thermometer?

The simplest way is to slowly rotate it between your fingers while holding it on the bottom and keeping it in the horizontal position. It may take a little practice, but you will soon be able to easily see the mercury column running down from the bulb. Simple read the number at the spot where the band of mercury ends. It is not necessary to be too exact—getting within one-half a degree is good enough. I would suggest that you become proficient in handling a thermometer before your baby ever gets sick. Take my word for it, this practice will save you a lot of trouble later on.

How accurate is a thermometer?

Our commerically available thermometers are quite accurate. However, there is one point I'd like to make about this. It has been shown that there may be variations of up to one-half degree from one thermometer to another. Therefore, it is sensible to use the same thermometer each time you take your baby's temperature.

What factors besides illness affect the baby's temperature?

1) The time of day: The temperature is usually lowest in the early morning and highest in the late afternoon or early evening. The average A.M. temperature is about 97° and by evening can be close to 100°.

2) Activity: This is most important. After vigorous exercise, including crying, a baby's temperature may go up one degree or maybe even more. This is why I recommend that whenever possible you take your baby's temperature after she has been at rest for a while. This reading will more accurately reflect her actual temperature and will give you a better idea as to whether or not she actually has fever.

3) Environmental temperature: An excessively hot house and/or overdressing your infant can easily push her temperature to 101° or higher.

I remember making a late-night house call. When I got into the apartment, it felt as if I had just walked into an oven. The windows were shut tight, and the steam was going full blast. To make matters worse, the sick baby was covered with layers of heavy clothing and hidden under a pile of blankets. His temperature was 105°. I opened the windows, had the heat turned down, got him out from under all the blankets, and took off his clothes. I then took the history from the mother and examined the baby. By this time about thirty minutes had elapsed. The temperature was taken again, and the thermometer now read 102.5°.

A final word of advice. Don't become a thermometer freak. Don't take your baby's temperature every time she sneezes. Don't take her temperature when she is well. The only time you should shake down your thermometer and use it is when you believe that your baby is sick.

FEVER

A rectal thermometer reading of over 100° F means fever. As I have explained, there is a normal range of temperature, roughly between 97° F and 100° F, and thus if your baby's temperature goes up beyond this range, he can be considered to have fever.

Fever is an important subject. Almost all parents will have to face the problem of a feverish baby sooner or later. Furthermore, there are all sorts of misconceptions about fever and what should be done about it. I should like to better prepare you for the time when your baby gets sick with an elevated temperature.

Let's start off by stating clearly that fever in itself is not harmful or dangerous to your baby. As a matter of fact, it can be extremely useful. Fever alerts us to the possibility of illness. This allows us to take action to find the *cause* of the fever, which is what is really important. Having your doctor track down the cause allows him to give the appropriate treatment.

Even though there is no reason to worry about fever,

parents do so anyway. Besides being concerned about what is causing the elevated temperature, they worry about the possibility of a fever convulsion. We'll cover this subject in the next chapter, but, very briefly, let me assure you that usually this type of seizure is not dangerous. It can readily be controlled and can often be prevented with appropriate management. Most important, febrile convulsions do not lead to brain damage.

Fever is *not* a disease. In almost all cases, fever is simply a sign that there is an infection somewhere in the body. It is nature's way of warning us that something is wrong. The elevated temperature response is one of the ways we react to the stress of a viral or bacterial infection. Fever also helps us keep track of how the illness is progressing. With these points in mind, there is no reason to be frightened by fever. Rather, it should be considered a normal body response to infection.

Should fever-reducing medications ever be used? There are two schools of thought about this, and I belong to the school that recommends using these medicines. If the temperature is allowed to rise too high, it increases the risk of a fever convulsion. Furthermore, a high temperature is uncomfortable for the baby and can interfere with his ability to sleep. It makes good sense to me to give a fever-reducing drug when your baby has a high fever, but it should not be given until you know the cause of the fever.

In my experience, the three most common signals of possible illness are (1) excessive fussiness and crankiness; (2) loss of appetite; and (3) restlessness. In such situations, I would suggest that you check your baby's temperature. Of course, if your baby feels unusually warm to the touch, it is also a good idea to take his temperature. If it turns out that your baby does have fever, my best advice is to then consult with your doctor. This should be done before you start any specific treatment on your own.

Many parents and grandparents believe that they don't need a thermometer. They tell me that they can determine whether or not the baby has a fever by simply feeling the skin. This method is really not that reliable. Many times a baby will actually feel cold to the touch when he has a fever, and conversely, he may feel quite warm but will turn out to have a perfectly normal temperature.

A study was carried out in the Good Samaritan Hospital in Phoenix, Arizona, on a large number of children. Almost one-half of the children who were judged to be without fever by palpation (done by nurse-assistants) actually had fever when thermometers were used. If you insist on feeling your child for evidence of fever, I would suggest that you feel the small of the back rather than the forehead. This will probably improve your chances of being correct. But by far the best method is to use a thermometer.

There is no rational reason to keep a baby with fever indoors. Let's put to rest, once and for all, the old wives' tale that taking a feverish baby out of the house is dangerous. This is utter nonsense. I certainly do not advise taking a sick child who has fever out in a blizzard, but I also don't think it's such a good idea when your baby is well. If your baby is not too sick and the weather outside is pleasant, it is perfectly okay to get out for some fresh air.

I will never forget making a house call to see a young child with the flu on one cold, windy January day. When I got into the apartment, it was freezing—the entire heating system had broken down the day before. Grandma lived two blocks away, so I asked why they had not taken the baby over there to take advantage of the more comfortable environment. The answer: "We were afraid to take the baby outside with his fever."

Let's now discuss the actual treatment of fever. As I've said before, the first and most important thing to do is to try to find out what is actually causing the fever. Certain infections need specific medication, and others do not. Your baby's physician should be called so that he can properly advise you. He may want to examine the baby or he may be able to take care of the problem over the phone, but he must be the one to make this decision. Your actual management of the fever itself is handled as follows:

1) **Feed your baby fluids:** Encourage your baby to drink, the more the better. Anything wet will do—water, tea, juice, or milk. This is very important in controlling fever.

2) **Keep your baby cool:** The baby is already too warm, so it makes little sense to cover him with heavy layers of clothing and a pile of thick blankets. It is helpful to cool off the house, turn down the heat, and open the windows. If you have air conditioning, by all means turn it on. Use a minimum of clothing.

3) **Employ fever-reducing medication:** The two most effective drugs for reducing fever (antipyretics) are aspirin and acetaminophen. You should check with your physician as to which he recommends and in what dosage. The usual and accepted aspirin dose, which may be given every four hours, is as follows:

6 months old	1/2 baby aspirin
1 year old	1 baby aspirin
2 years old	2 baby aspirins

I would not recommend that you wake your baby in order to give him a fever-reducing medicine unless your doctor specifically tells you to do so. Instead, let him sleep—he needs the rest. You can be sure that if he gets hot enough, he will wake up by himself.

4) **Sponging and bathing:** If your baby's temperature is very high (above 104°F), I advise you to take off all his clothing and gently sponge him by wetting your hand or a towel in lukewarm water and rubbing his arms, legs, and back. This sponging increases evaporation and helps lower the temperature. If the fever is extremely high, you can sponge with cold water or with water and rubbing alcohol mixed in equal parts. However, this method of

external cooling may cause shivering. Since shivering increases muscular activity and oxygen demand, it may actually contribute to raising the temperature. If the sponging causes the baby to shiver, you should immediately stop. Another very effective way to lower temperature is to immerse the baby into a cool water bath.

These methods of fever reduction should be used if the fever is very high, especially if your baby has had a previous fever convulsion. It is important not to allow the temperature to rise to the level that would trigger another convulsion.

Remember, there is never any reason to panic when your baby has fever. By following the suggestions that I have outlined, you should be able to calmly and effectively handle the situation. Relax, shake down your thermometer, and carry on.

FEVER CONVULSIONS

Let's begin by defining our terms. We will be describing the type of convulsion that is caused by high fever. This is called a fever convulsion or febrile seizure. (Fever and febrile are synonymous, and convulsion and seizure are synonymous.) This elevated temperature is due to an infection anywhere in the body that does not primarily involve the brain. As a rule, this type of convulsion is not in itself dangerous. It does not damage the child in any way.

Fever is by far the most common cause of all convulsions in infants and children. Since this type of convulsion occurs with relative frequency, it is important for parents to understand what is going on and to learn to handle the problem if and when it develops.

There is nothing more frightening to new parents than the thought that their baby might have a convulsion and that this convulsion may cause brain damage. This is just not so. Many parents also believe that a convulsion means epilepsy and that epilepsy leads to mental retardation.

This is absolutely untrue. The sooner we put to rest these false associations, the better.

Any type of infection, viral or bacterial, can bring on the fever that leads to the seizure. This febrile convulsion is *not* epilepsy. Epilepsy refers to a condition, seen much less often, in which convulsions occur *without* fever. Therefore, by definition, the child who has fever during a seizure does not have epilepsy. Again, febrile convulsions do not cause brain damage and do not lead to mental retardation.

How does the high fever cause a convulsion?

Each and every infant and child has her own "threshold convulsion temperature." This refers to the specific temperature at which the baby will have a convulsion—the specific temperature at which her brain will become irritated enough by fever to trigger a seizure. This temperature reading varies from child to child. For example, one baby may have a seizure every time her temperature reaches 103°, and another one will not convulse until her temperature hits 104°. Yet another child may have a threshold of 106°; her chances of ever having a convulsion are quite low, since the temperature of most infants and children never reaches so high a level. According to various studies, the average temperature at which a febrile seizure occurs is 104°.

It should be a source of comfort for you to know that the great majority of infants and children never have a febrile seizure. This group has high threshold convulsion temperatures and is fortunate enough never to reach the magic number. Or they may be lucky enough never to contract any infection that causes a particularly high temperature. The specific cause of the fever is not related to the development of a seizure—the only significant factor is the "threshold." If this threshold is reached, a seizure results. If a baby has had a fever convulsion at 104°, the chances are good that if during another illness her temperature again reaches 104°, she will have another seizure.

A number of separate investigations have shown that 2 to 3 percent of all children suffer fever convulsions. In the United States this figure represents 500,000 youngsters. The first seizure usually occurs between six months and three years of age, with the greatest number occurring between one and two years of age. As the child grows older, the incidence of seizures decreases. Febrile convulsions are rarely seen after nine years of age.

Febrile seizures often run in families. In eliciting a careful history from the parents of a child who has had one, I frequently find that one of the parents or a brother or sister also has had fever convulsions. Of course, this does not always hold true. As a matter of fact, the last three children I've treated for this all had negative family histories.

There is another widely held misconception, namely, that a child who has had fever convulsions will develop epilepsy later on. While it is true that this can occur, in the overwhelming majority of cases it just does not happen. Proof of this is that 97 percent of all children under five who have had febrile seizures are completely free of convulsions in later life.

In almost all cases the fever convulsion will occur during the first day of the illness. Another point to keep in mind is that there is usually only one convulsion during an illness. What is the usual story? A one- or two-year-old becomes ill, often with a sore throat or ear infection, and starts to run a high temperature. When the temperature reaches her "threshold for convulsion," there is a seizure. She may start to twitch and then shake violently all over. She loses consciousness, her eyes rolling back, and she often will foam at the mouth. These generalized convulsions caused by the fever rarely last longer than five minutes, and they stop without specific treatment. The child then usually goes off to sleep, and when she wakes up, she is fine. The first seizure is always a harrowing and frightening experience to the parents, but you must remember that no permanent brain damage results and your baby will be as good as new when it's all over.

What should be done if your child suddenly has her first febrile convulsion?

First of all, remain calm—screaming and hysterics don't help at all. The most important thing to do is to prevent your child from hurting herself during the seizure. Place her on her stomach with her head turned to one side. Remove anything she may have in her mouth. If she appears to be biting her tongue, keep her jaws separated with the end of a pen, a clothespin, or your fingers wrapped in a handkerchief. Make sure that she does not bang her head on a hard surface. The next step is to call your doctor. By the time you reach him and certainly by the time he gets to see the child, the seizure will probably be over. Nonetheless, it is most important that she be examined. The cause of the fever must be determined so that proper treatment can be started. Some types of infection require a specific medication, and the earlier the diagnosis is made, the better. The convulsion may have actually been caused by an infection of the brain, and this is a medical emergency—treatment must be instituted immediately. If your physician is not available, take the child to the emergency room of the nearest hospital so that another doctor can examine her. If your own doctor is on his way over, the next step is to reduce the child's temperature. Take off her clothing and cool off the room as much as possible. Then gently sponge her by wetting your hand or towel in tepid (lukewarm) water and rubbing arms, legs, and back. This sponging increases the baby's evaporation, and this lowers the temperature. If the fever is exceptionally high, sponging with cold water or with water and alcohol mixed in equal parts may be carried out, but you must be careful not to do so too vigorously. This can cause shivering, which in itself raises the temperature. Another effective method is to immerse the child in a cool water bath for a few minutes. A fever-reducing medicine such as aspirin or acetaminophen should be given. If the child is unable to take medication by mouth, aspirin can be given by suppository. As a general rule, a one-year-old gets a 2 1/2-grain suppository and a two- to five-year-old a 5-grain suppository. I would advise against the use of cold water enemas to reduce fever, since this method has been shown to be dangerous.

Can anything be done to prevent the first febrile convulsion?

Obviously the answer is to never allow your child's temperature to reach her particular threshold. Unfortunately, this can't always be done. There is no way to determine this critical temperature before the first seizure, but if you start measures to lower your child's high fever early in an illness, the chances will be better that the temperature will not rise high enough to trigger the convulsion. With any febrile illness, it is most important to encourage your baby to drink plenty of fluids, such as water, tea, or juice. This will go a long way toward lowering the temperature. Keep her cool and keep her room cool. An antipyretic (fever reducer) should be given. Aspirin or acetaminophen in proper dosage are the two most effective drugs available. Your doctor should be consulted so that he may determine the cause of the fever and what type of treatment might be needed. If the temperature continues to climb, sponging (previously described) should be begun. This approach to fever will often prevent the temperature from reaching the threshold, and so there will be no convulsion.

What can be done to prevent further fever seizures?

This is one of the areas of pediatrics in which there is a real difference of opinion. This controversy relates to the use of phenobarbital. Some doctors recommend that any child who has had a febrile seizure should be kept on daily doses of phenobarbital for a period of two seizure-free years. If the child is less than three years old at the onset, the phenobarbital should be given until the patient is five years old. Other physicians do not agree with this approach. They believe that phenobarbital should be kept in the house and used only when the susceptible child develops fever; it should not be used continually while the baby is well. In my experience, both methods are effective in cutting down the chances of another febrile convulsion. Your physician will decide both how the phenobarbital should be used and the proper dose of the medication. In addition to the phenobarbital, the key to the prevention of further fever convulsions is not to allow the temperature to reach the threshold of the first convulsion. This requires the prompt fever-reducing measures we have suggested.

To summarize:

1) Febrile convulsions are not dangerous and stop by themselves without specific treatment.

2) A febrile seizure is not epilepsy, and it does not cause brain damage.

3) Keep calm and prevent your child from injuring herself during the convulsion.

4) Treat the fever with antipyretics, fluids, sponging, and a cool environment.

5) Add phenobarbital to the fever-reducing routine if your child is susceptible to fever convulsions.

6) Notify your doctor if a fever convulsion occurs.

THE COMMON COLD

The cold is by far the most common illness of infancy and childhood. New parents become concerned when their baby catches a cold, and the younger the infant affected, the greater the worry. There are all sorts of misconceptions and old wives' tales associated with colds. I'll try to put them to rest once and for all. Unnecessary worrying can be avoided by learning the facts and unlearning the myths. I want you to be able to calmly and confidently handle the situation when your baby gets his first (or next) cold.

A cold is a virus infection that causes an inflammation of the linings of the nose, throat, and larynx (voice box). This results in swelling and the outpouring of fluid and mucus. Another name for the common cold is an upper respiratory infection (URI). I will be using the cold and URI interchangeably as we go along.

At last count, well over one hundred different viruses had been isolated and implicated as causing a cold. Therefore, it is obvious that a URI is not a single disease entity. Rather, it is a syndrome characterized by similar features.

The main characteristic of a URI is the outpouring of fluid and mucus from the inflamed linings of the nose and throat. This produces a runny nose and watery eyes. Some of the fluid and mucus also runs down the throat. The nasal discharge starts by being watery and often becomes thick and yellow as the cold progresses. The nose may become plugged up by this thick mucus, and this can cause the baby to breathe noisily. A baby with a cold usually becomes irritable because the mucus irritates her throat. There frequently is accompanying fever, listlessness, and loss of appetite. As the cold progresses, the baby begins to cough. The cough further irritates the tissues and causes additional coughing, and a vicious cycle is started. The average URI lasts between seven and ten days.

Fever is usually low-grade if the infant with a cold is under three months old. Between three months and three years of age, the fever of the cold is usually higher. I might add that the fever of an uncomplicated URI usually lasts about three days. The younger infant usually does some vomiting. This is due to his stomach's becoming irritated by swallowed mucus. Diarrhea is also more common in the younger infant with a cold.

The question as to exactly how a baby catches a cold always comes up. The answer is that he simply catches it from somebody else around him with a URI. A URI is very contagious and may be spread easily, especially during the first two or three days of the illness. It is mainly transmitted via "droplet" spray—by coughing or sneezing. It may also be spread by breathing into the face or by kissing on the mouth. A baby does not catch a cold by going outside the house or by being in a draft or by his blanket's falling off or by not being dressed warmly enough (despite what Grandma may say).

It is interesting that some babies catch a cold and

others do not when similarly exposed. The explanation for this lies in the resistance of the particular infant at the time of the contact. Teething and fatigue may lower an infant's resistance and make him more susceptible to picking up the infection if and when he is exposed to it.

Most colds occur between September and April. The explanation for this is unclear. Perhaps during the winter months there is more close contact with people, since more time is spent indoors. But babies can catch colds anytime.

A newborn is not immune to a URI. The mother does not transfer any URI immunity to the child during the pregnancy. This is unlike measles, for example. If the new mother has had measles in the past, she transfers immunity to measles to her newborn baby, and this immunity lasts for approximately the first six months of life. But there is no such thing when it comes to a URI.

The incubation period of the common cold is usually three to seven days. By incubation period we mean the time between exposure to the virus and the development of the signs and symptoms of the cold.

Both allergy and teething can mimic the signs and symptoms of a cold. If the baby is allergic to milk or to a particular food or to something in the environment such as dust or pollen, he may develop a nasal allergy (allergic rhinitis). In such a case, there is a profuse, watery, clear discharge from the nose which continues for many days or even weeks. This is often associated with excessive tearing of the eyes. During the teething process the baby salivates more than usual, and this drooling may also be mistaken for a cold.

There is no reason to stop bathing a baby with an uncomplicated cold. As a matter of fact, a bath can be helpful in soothing the baby and making him more comfortable. Just remember to dry him thoroughly after the bath.

During the course of a URI, most babies sneeze more

often than usual. This is okay, and nothing need be done to try to stop the sneezing. It is the body's way of getting rid of extra mucus.

Babies are very susceptible to colds. In my experience, the average younger child has four or five colds a year. I might add that the child in his first year of school (the nursery school or kindergarten) is notorious for the large number of colds he acquires. During this first year away from home, the child is exposed to many more children than ever before. Therefore, his risk of coming into contact with one of the viruses causing a URI is markedly increased. And when he comes home from school with his newly acquired cold, he promptly and easily passes it on to his younger brother or sister.

Let me state as forcefully as possible that there is no specific cure for a cold. So-called cold vaccines are worthless. There is no solid scientific evidence proving that high doses of vitamin C either prevent or cure the cold. The best we can do is to help relieve the symptoms of the cold while allowing it to run its natural course. Let's go over this step by step.

1) **Fever:** Fever should be treated with the appropriate dose of a fever-reducing medication, such as aspirin or acetaminophen.

2) **Runny nose:** Nose drops or an oral decongestant can be used, after consulting with your baby's physician. Suctioning the fluid and mucus from the nose with a nasal syringe can be quite effective. A good method to follow is to let gravity help to drain the mucus foward from the back of the throat and the back of the nose so that the nasal syringe can suck it out more easily. This is done by tilting the baby's head downward at a slight angle (as over the side of the crib) for a few minutes before using the syringe. You should remember that up to nine months of age, infants breathe primarily through their noses and not through their mouths; therefore, it is important to try to keep their nasal passages clear. A word of caution: nose

drops should never be used continually for long periods of time. A rebound phenomenon may result after prolonged use which can cause even more swollen nasal passages.

3) **Cough:** A cough preparation in the proper dosage can be given—after discussion with your baby's doctor.

4) **Fluids:** It is always a good idea to increase the fluid intake of the infant or child who has a cold. Water, tea, and juice are all fine for this purpose.

5) **Solid Foods:** Since the baby's appetite is usually reduced when he has a cold, it is important not to try to force solids down if the baby refuses them. All this will do is cause the infant to vomit.

6) **Environment:** The baby can be kept comfortable by keeping the house cool. If the weather is good, the baby should be taken outside for some fresh air. There is no reason to keep a baby with a cold in the house. Increasing the humidity in the house can also be helpful. This is done by using a vaporizer or a humidifier which will soothe the inflamed tissues of the nose and throat and will help reduce the cough.

Colds cannot be prevented. There is no magic drug available and no immunization against it. When you realize that each of over one hundred different viruses can cause a cold, you can understand how difficult it would be to develop a vaccine against the URI. Since babies catch colds from contact with somebody else who has a cold, it makes good sense to try (within reason) to avoid exposing the infant unduly. He certainly cannot and should not be kept in a glass cage, but you should try to avoid large crowds. It is also wise to screen your visitors, especially other young children with cold symptoms. If there is no way to keep them out of your house, at least make sure that they don't get too close to the baby.

If the irritation and inflammation spread beyond the nose and throat to the trachea (windpipe), lungs, or ears, complications result. Among the more common complications of a cold are bronchitis, pneumonia, and ear infections. When the body's natural defenses are weakened by fighting off the virus infection, these so-called secondary bacterial infections occur. Signs of such an infection are high fever, severe cough, and very pained crying. Other associated findings which may point to complications are rapid breathing, difficulty in breathing, or swollen glands in the neck. It is a fact that younger babies are more susceptible to the complications of a cold than the older child because there is a shorter distance between the nose, ears, and throat in the baby than there is in the older child.

Your doctor should be called to answer any questions you may have about the management of the ordinary cold. He certainly must be consulted when you think that you are dealing with more than the usual cold and especially when you suspect that the baby may have developed a secondary complication. Your doctor may wish to see the baby, or he may prescribe medication over the phone. The use of an antibiotic is indicated if your baby shows signs and symptoms of a secondary complication such as bronchitis or an ear infection.

With a bit of experience, a great majority of URIs can be handled by the parents alone. Babies are strong and resilient, and if given a bit of help, they recover from their colds smoothly and rapidly. Simply stock up with a good supply of tissues and stop worrying.

BREATH HOLDING

Breath-holding episodes are harmless. They do not hurt your baby in any way. But the first time your baby holds her breath can be a very frightening experience. Many new parents are unfamiliar with this common condition, and I should like to discuss it with you in some detail.

The usual sequence of events is as follows: During a period of vigorous crying, the baby who is breathing rapidly suddenly stops her respirations. During this period of apnea (no breathing), she can turn pale or blue and may even become stiff and rigid. If the episode of breath holding lasts long enough, there is a momentary loss of consciousness, during which the baby may twitch or actually convulse. Immediately after losing consciousness, the baby *always* starts to breathe spontaneously, her normal color returns, and she stops convulsing.

Following the episode, she is fine or just a bit pale for a few minutes, and sometimes she goes to sleep. After she awakens from this sleep, she is perfectly normal in every way. Most of these breath-holding episodes stop by themselves before the baby loses consciousness. A few stop only after unconsciousness, but, most important, they all always stop and no damage ever results.

During these episodes the child voluntarily stops breathing, and so less oxygen gets to the brain. If this period of anoxia (lack of oxygen) lasts long enough, it leads to unconsciousness. After losing consciousness, the child no longer has voluntary control of her breathing; so her respirations immediately start up again and all is well.

The usual provocations for breath holding are pain, fear, or anger. It usually happens during a temper tantrum, after a painful injury, or after the baby is frightened or surprised. In other words, anything that will cause the baby to cry vigorously can trigger it. There is nothing you can do to prevent these troublesome episodes.

Most frequently, babies between the ages of six and eighteen months are affected. It can start as early as three months of age and may continue until the child is five or six years old. It is rarely seen after the age of six. It is also rare for breath holding to begin after three years of age. We just don't know why some babies are breath-holders and others are not.

The incidence of breath holding has not been clearly determined. In one study of a clinic population in Baltimore, about one-half of the children were breath-holders. I myself have not seen it quite that often. The incidence in which the breath holder actually passes out is, of course, much lower. Breath holding is not necessarily associated with behavior problems. In my experience, breath-holders do not have greater emotional or psychological problems than the nonbreath-holders. I have noticed that active, energetic infants more commonly hold their breaths than calmer, more placid babies. Breath holding does not cause brain damage, and it is not related to mental retardation. It is not a form of epilepsy. Occasionally, it may be difficult to differentiate between a breath-holding spell and a real seizure disorder. There is a problem in diagnosis with breath-holding episodes that result in loss of consciousness followed by twitching or shaking. Your baby's doctor will determine whether it is simply breath holding or a seizure disorder. If you have any doubt in your mind, by all means consult your physician.

During a breath-holding episode the main thing to do is to remain clam. I realize this won't be easy for you, especially the first time it happens. It is not necessary to do anything to try to snap the baby out of it. The common practice of throwing water in the baby's face is probably useless. It is important to display an attitude of unconcern during the breath-holding periods so that the child will not purposely use this technique as a weapon to dominate the family. I have seen this happen over and over again, especially with two-year-olds. The youngster, realizing how upset and frightened her parents become, simply holds her breath every time she is frustrated in any way. She uses her breath holding as a sword over her parents' heads. On the other hand, if the child is made to realize that she does not gain anything by holding her breath and that you are not upset by it, the habit disappears much more rapidly.

Some studies have shown that in about one-third of the cases of breath-holders, there is a positive family history. I personally have not seen this in my practice, and I do not think that this is so.

There is no known relationship between breath holding and illness. The only possible exception may be related to anemia. Some investigations have demonstrated an association between breath holding and anemia. It is believed by some that anemia somehow predisposes a baby to breath holding. I have not myself been impressed with this line of reasoning. However, since there is a question, it makes good sense to have the baby checked for anemia if she is a habitual breath-holder. If she is found to be anemic, she can be treated with the appropriate medication as prescribed by your doctor.

The number of breath-holding episodes varies from baby to baby. Some may have one breath-holding episode and never have another. Others may have a number of breath-holding episodes each day. It is important to remember that the number of breath-holding episodes is not significant. Even if she has many every day, they will not do any damage.

In summary, breath-holding episodes are harmless and do not lead to any future difficulty. It is important to be able to recognize these frightening occurrences for what they are. They sometimes need to be differentiated from a true seizure disorder. Once the diagnosis of breath holding is made, there is no longer any reason for you to worry. Ignore the whole thing. It will stop in due course without treatment.

HEAD INJURIES

My telephone rings. "Dr. Eden, my baby just fell off the dressing table and hit her head on the floor. What should I do?"

This is an important problem that most parents will have to face sooner or later. When it happens, it can be terribly frightening. As a practicing pediatrician for over twenty years, I know that many mothers and fathers are unprepared to handle this situation. Very often they worry unnecessarily. More important, they sometimes react too little and too late.

Head injuries can be divided into three broad categories, each of which requires a different approach on your part.

1) **Mild:** Nothing needs to be done except to carefully observe the baby.

2) **Moderate:** This requires an immediate call to your child's doctor.

3) **Severe:** This is an emergency, and immediate hospitalization is necessary.

In most cases, it will not be too difficult for you to determine the type of head injury your baby has received. Occasionally, there is some overlap. Of course, if you have any question about it, it makes good sense to consult with you doctor, just to be on the safe side.

1) **Mild:** This is by far the most common type of childhood head injury. The baby falls, hits his head, cries for a few minutes, and then resumes his normal activities. There is no vomiting, loss of consciousness, or change in his color. He looks and acts just fine right after the accident.

If this is the type of injury your baby sustains, there is very little for you to worry about. No specific action need be taken except to watch him carefully for the next forty-eight hours for any change in his normal behavior pattern, especially increasing drowsiness and lethargy. If nothing unusual happens during this forty-eight-hour period, you can forget about it.

If the injury caused the skin to be broken, the area should be cleaned with an antiseptic. Any deep cut or laceration may require suturing, and in such cases your doctor should be notified. If you notice some swelling at the site of the injury, cold compresses should be applied.

2) **Moderate:** This refers to a head injury that is associated with a concussion (meaning a brief loss of consciousness followed by complete recovery) or with vomiting immediately after the accident. Although the great majority of these moderate head injuries turn out to be perfectly harmless, your doctor must always be called. He may want to examine the baby or he may have you observe him at home, but this decision must be made by the physician and not by you. When talking to your doctor, it is important that you tell him exactly how the accident occurred. There is an obvious difference between a baby sitting on a thick rug and falling forward on his forehead and a baby dropping head first from the bathroom sink to the tile floor.

HEAD INJURIES

3) **Severe:** This is a head injury in which the baby is knocked unconscious and remains unconscious. This is a medical emergency and requires immediate hospitalization. Place the baby on his side with his head slightly elevated and transport him in this position to the hospital. Other signs pointing to a severe head injury are persistent vomiting, convulsions, irregular breathing, pale color, and bleeding from the ear canal. Faced with any of these, you must take the baby to the hospital at once. In my experience, it is rare for a baby to sustain this type of severe head injury from the ordinary household accident. It does occur, however, in automobile accidents.

Any baby with a head injury who is kept at home must be observed carefully for the following forty-eight hours. The greatest danger following any head injury is bleeding within the brain. The signs that may indicate this type of bleeding are

1) Persistent vomiting
2) Unequal eye pupil size
3) Excessive drowsiness and increasing lethargy (most important)
4) Weakness of one arm or one leg
5) Continuous crying
6) Any change in color from normal to pale

If you notice any of these signs or symptoms, call your doctor immediately. I would also advise that you wake the baby two separate times during the first night following the accident to make sure that he is sleeping normally and that he has not lapsed into unconsciousness. This is especially important following the moderate type of head injury.

There is one additional problem that you must be aware of if your baby has had either a moderate or severe head injury. In rare cases, a blood clot may gradually accumulate under the skull ("chronic subdural clot"), and there is a long delay after the accident, sometimes up to one month, before signs of increasing drowsiness or loss of balance develop. If this does happen, the baby must be taken straight to the hospital.

There is no way to prevent your baby from ever banging his head on some hard surface. You must not feel guilty every time he hits his head on something or other. Normal babies are active, and they move rapidly. Reasonable precautions should be taken to try to prevent serious injuries. It makes little sense to leave a nine-month-old on the kitchen table while you go to answer the telephone. This particular example comes to mind since it actually happened to one of my patients. Luckily, the baby landed on his backside rather than on his head. So the little fellow ended up with an ache in a much less vulnerable area than his brain. But it is wrong to be so worried and overprotective that it interferes with the baby's normal movements and explorations.

The important thing is to be aware of the danger signs following the head injuries. If there is *any doubt in your mind*, your baby's doctor must be immediately notified. The law of averages is on your side: serious head injuries are relatively rare. But a few are real emergencies, and in these cases no time should be lost in getting the baby to a doctor.

With the knowledge of these danger signals firmly in mind, you should be able to relax a bit and not worry about every little insignificant knock to your baby's skull. It is amazing how remarkably resilient a child's head is to the numerous bangs it receives during the course of a normal childhood.

JAUNDICE IN THE NEWBORN

Jaundice is the condition in which a yellow bile pigment called *bilirubin*, carried in the blood, is deposited into the skin, mucus membranes, and sclera (white of the eye). This results in these areas' becoming stained yellow. It follows that anything causing a significant increase in the amount of bilirubin in the blood will lead to jaundice.

Since jaundice is so common in the newborn, many parents must face it. About half of all healthy full-term newborns become slightly jaundiced, usually on the third or fourth day of life. This subject is poorly understood by the majority of new mothers and fathers.

I will never forget a midnight phone call from the mother of a three-day-old infant still in the hospital: "This morning my doctor told me that my baby was jaundiced but not to worry about it. I am frantic. Could you please examine my baby? Will she die from liver disease?" Everything turned out fine. The newborn was only slightly jaundiced, and the jaundice did in fact clear up rapidly. The only mistake made was that the physician did not adequately explain what was going on to the mother. Parents are entitled to full and complete explanations, and sometimes we physicians just do not take the time to give them.

Bilirubin is the end product of the breakdown of red blood cells (actually a breakdown of the oxygen-carrying red pigment called *hemoglobin* in the red blood cell). Normally, red blood cells break down slowly and steadily as they get older, and the bilirubin that is thereby released is carried in the blood to the liver. In the liver a process called *conjugation* takes place which allows the bilirubin to be excreted from the body through the intestine and out in the stool. If the red blood cells break down at a normal rate and if the liver works efficiently, bilirubin cannot accumulate in the blood, and jaundice does not develop. But if the newborn's red blood cells break down too rapidly, the liver is immature, or there is a combination of both factors present, jaundice is bound to occur.

As I stated earlier, jaundice is quite common in the newborn baby. In non-Caucasian babies it may be missed unless you look at the whites of their eyes. In the case of premature babies, the incidence of jaundice is even higher. There is a big difference between the jaundice seen in the newborn and the jaundice of an older child or adult. This difference is related to the usual causes of the jaundice. The two most common causes of jaundice in the newborn are so-called physiologic jaundice and blood group incompatibilities; rarely is the jaundice due to liver disease or obstruction. On the other hand, the jaundice seen in older children and adults is usually caused by liver disease (hepatitis) or by some form of obstruction preventing the bilirubin from passing through the intestine.

Physiologic jaundice is the common condition in which the newborn's skin and sclera become yellow starting around the third day of life and which usually disappears by one week of age. Physiologic jaundice is harmless and does not usually require any treatment. It is by far the most frequent cause of jaundice in the newborn. There are a number of different mechanisms to explain why this occurs. The main cause is simply that during the first few days of life the newborn's liver is immature and does not work very efficiently. As the bilirubin reaches the liver of the newborn, there is a deficiency of a certain liver enzyme that prevents the liver from doing the conjugating job properly. This immature liver just cannot handle all the bilirubin coming through. The bilirubin that is not conjugated cannot be excreted into the intestine and builds up in the bloodstream and stains the skin yellow. As the liver of the normal newborn becomes more efficient and as the body manufactures more and more of the missing enzyme, the conjugation process is performed appropriately, and the jaundice rapidly disappears. In the case of the premature newborn, the liver is even more immature, and so it is not surprising that a still higher percentage develop physiologic jaundice. It may take from three to four weeks for the jaundice to disappear, since the premature's liver often takes that long to reach maximum efficiency. The main point to remember about physiologic jaundice is that it is not a disease and does not damage your baby.

Jaundice itself is not dangerous to the newborn unless it becomes very severe. If too much bilirubin accumulates in the blood, there is the danger of brain damage. This damage is caused by the large amounts of bilirubin in the blood staining the brain cells and is called *kernicterus*. Unfortunately, once these brain cells are affected, the damage is irreversible; so you can see how important it is that the bilirubin levels in the blood not be allowed to rise too high.

Kernicterus develops when the bilirubin level in the blood of the newborn rises above a certain dangerous level. In the case of a premature or sick newborn, this danger level is lower than in a full-term, healthy baby. The sick newborn and the premature newborn are more susceptible and at greater risk to the possibility of developing kernicterus than a healthy, full-term newborn. Therefore, the jaundice in these groups must be treated earlier and more vigorously.

Kernicterus can be prevented by prompt treatment. With the two methods currently available that lower the bilirubin level, we can prevent brain damage that develops from too much jaundice. These methods are (1) exchange transfusion and (2) phototherapy.

Exchange transfusion is simply the step-by-step mechanical removal of all of the baby's blood supply and replacement with fresh blood.

Phototherapy means placing the infant under a high-intensity light source. Light has been shown to break down the bilirubin and, therefore, lower the level in the blood. Your infant's doctor will use these forms of treatment if and when they are indicated. These procedures are reserved for the more severe forms of jaundice and are not usually used to treat physiologic jaundice.

The most common cause of severe jaundice in the full-term newborn is blood group incompatibilities. When there is a conflict between the blood of the mother and the blood of the baby, the infant's red blood cells can be broken down more rapidly than normal (this process is called *hemolysis*). As a result of this rapid hemolysis, large amounts of bilirubin are released into the blood, the immature liver of the newborn cannot take care of the increased load, and so jaundice develops. The two main types of blood group incompatibility are (1) Rh incompatibility and (2) ABO incompatibility.

In Rh incompatibility the mother is Rh-negative and the father is Rh-positive. If the newborn is Rh-positive, a resulting blood group incompatibility is possible. Statistically, 12 percent of married couples have the setup for Rh incompatibility, but, in point of fact, only one in two hundred babies is affected. This means that most of the time, despite the proper setup, the newborn does not have any trouble. It should be added that Rh incompatibility seldom occurs with the firstborn baby.

In ABO incompatibility, the mother is type O and the baby is either type A or type B. This condition sometimes causes hemolysis of the baby's red blood cells. ABO incompatibility is often seen in first babies but usually does not cause as severe a degree of jaundice as we see in the Rh incompatibilities.

If the blood group incompatibility is severe enough to cause a good deal of jaundice, the affected baby is treated either by exchange transfusion or by phototherapy, and at times by both methods. These treatments are most effective, and the results by and large are excellent.

There are many other less common causes of jaundice in the newborn. These include certain types of infection and certain drugs. Your doctor's job is to track down the specific cause and treat accordingly.

Suffice to say, it is very important for the nurses and physicians to examine and observe all newborns very carefully for the development of jaundice. If this jaundice occurs within the first twenty-four hours of life, it usually means that there is some trouble. Appropriate tests must be carried out to determine the cause so that the baby can be properly treated. If the jaundice develops when the baby is two or three days old, it almost always means physiologic jaundice. And I repeat, this condition is harmless.

The two main points to be remembered are (1) jaundice may be a sign of many disorders, and so it can never be ignored; and (2) the level of bilirubin in the blood must never be allowed to reach a dangerously high level which might cause brain damage.

It is very difficult to determine if there is jaundice when looking at the baby under an artificial light source. Daylight observation makes it much easier. In order for us to be able to see jaundice of the skin, the bilirubin level has to reach a level of about 6 to 7 milligrams percent. This level of bilirubin is very safe. Only when the bilirubin level rises to close to 20 milligrams percent do we really have to worry. The exact level of bilirubin is determined by a simple blood test. All hospital laboratories are equipped to perform this test. If the newborn is healthy, sucking well, and thriving, there is no blood group incompatibility, and if she is only slightly jaundiced, this jaundice is almost certainly physiologic. Obviously, if a baby is taken home from the hospital with slight jaundice or with no jaundice at all and then later on turns yellower, your doctor must be consulted immediately.

There is one other cause of jaundice in the newborn, and that is breast milk. One in two hundred breast-fed babies become jaundiced. This is due to a certain substance found in the breast milk of a few mothers that inhibits or stops the liver from conjugating bilirubin. This substance slows down the production of the specific liver enzyme that is so important in the conjugation process. This type of jaundice usually develops during the second week of life. The important thing to remember is that this form of jaundice does not become severe enough to damage the infant. Actually, if the breast-feeding is stopped for two or three days, the jaundice clears up rapidly. Breast-feeding may then be started again and the jaundice does not recur.

In the great majority of cases, the newborn's jaundice is harmless and self-limiting. After the jaundice has cleared there is no residual damage to the baby. The more severe form of newborn jaundice usually means a blood group incompatibility. Small prematures and acutely ill newborns are more susceptible to jaundice. With the current methods available to us, all these infants can be treated quite satisfactorily so that brain damage is prevented.

Now that you better understand what it's all about, there is no reason to be frightened if your new baby develops some jaundice while in the hospital nursery.

Answers to Questions Mothers Most Frequently Ask

QUESTIONS AND ANSWERS

My baby is nine months old and does not have a single tooth in his mouth. Is this anything to worry about?

No, there is absolutely nothing to be concerned about. There is great variation in the time the first tooth appears. On the average, the first tooth comes in at around six to seven months of age, but some babies already have teeth by three months of age, and others have no teeth until after their first birthday. There is no correlation between intelligence or overall general development and the age the first tooth appears.

My neighbor just told me that she thinks my newborn baby is tongue-tied. What should I do about this?

By all means have your baby's doctor check this out. In all probability you have nothing to worry about. Let me explain a little about this subject. There is a little band of tissue called the *frenum* that binds the tongue down to the floor of the mouth. Occasionally, the frenum may interfere with the free protrusion of the tongue. In such cases, you may notice a notch at the tip of the tongue. Usually, the frenum stretches with time, and so nothing need be done. Contrary to what you may have heard, this condition does not cause speech problems later on. Rarely, the frenum must be cut in order to loosen the tongue. This is a relatively simple office procedure.

My baby has a strawberry-colored, raised area on the back of his neck. What is it and what should I do about it?

It sounds as if your baby has what is called a *hemangioma*. These hemangiomas, or birthmarks, usually appear after birth and enlarge rapidly during the first year of life. They are raised, a reddish-strawberry in color, and soft in consistency. Almost all of them disappear completely by three years of age if they are left alone. It is unnecessary to treat hemangiomas with dry ice or acid or some other caustic substance. Such a procedure may actually result in permanent scarring. Rarely is surgery necessary to remove the hemangioma. Show it to your baby's doctor. I have seen many large birthmarks of this type, and without exception, they all completely disappeared before the child started school.

I have just been told by my doctor that my baby boy has a hydrocele and that I shouldn't worry about it. What do you think?

I agree with your doctor. Hydroceles are very common in baby boys and almost always disappear by themselves. A hydrocele is a water sac around the testicle. It can develop on one side or on both sides. Most disappear by the time the baby is one year old. They are not painful, no matter how large they may be. Hydroceles often change in size as they fill and empty with water. Occasionally, a hydrocele may be associated with an inguinal hernia; so they should be observed carefully. Inguinal hernias appear as small, round lumps in the groin on one or both sides. If you notice one of these lumps, your doctor should be immediately notified. Whereas nothing need be done for a hydrocele, an inguinal hernia requires surgical repair.

I can feel only one testicle in my baby's scrotal sac. Is this normal?

Your doctor should be consulted about this. If one of your baby's testicles is truly undescended, it is important that he know about it. Very often what you may believe is an undescended testicle is simply what we call a retractile testicle. This is a testicle that moves up and down and in all cases finally comes down permanently. No treatment is necessary for a retractile testicle. If your baby's scrotum or sac appears "lived in"—in other words, if there is a normal-sized scrotum—the chances are that you are not dealing with a true undescended testicle. But, as I said before, your doctor must be the one to decide if your baby has an undescended or a retractile testicle.

I am two months pregnant and a heavy cigarette smoker. I have been told that this may cause harm to my baby. Is this true?

My answer is an emphatic yes. This is an extremely important subject and deserves some discussion beyond that simple "yes." Many studies have clearly shown that heavy cigarette smoking by women during their pregnancies results in smaller-sized babies than for women who never smoke or gave up smoking during the pregnancy. Further, heavy cigarette smoking during pregnancy actually decreases the fetal breathing movements, and these breathing movements are an index of the fetus's well-being. A recent investigation carried out in New Zealand found that the IQ of children of women who smoked during pregnancy was significantly lower than that of a comparable group whose mothers did not smoke. For all these reasons, I would strongly recommend that you stop or at least cut down on your cigarette consumption during your pregnancy. There is no question that heavy cigarette smoking by the pregnant woman is a definite risk for the developing fetus.

Although you have not asked, there is another danger for your child related to your cigarette smoking. A recent study conducted in Israel showed many more hospital admissions due to bronchitis and pneumonia during the first year of life in babies whose parents were heavy cigarette smokers than in the group of babies whose parents did not smoke. Similar results were reported in another investigation from London. In other words, heavy cigarette smoking in the house during the first year of a baby's life makes it more likely that he will end up in the hospital with a severe respiratory infection.

Evidence has accumulated clearly demonstrating that the children of cigarette-smoking parents start smoking earlier and smoke more frequently than those raised by nonsmoking parents. Our children learn by example. We all should know by now the devastating effects of cigarette smoking; so why tempt the fates as far as our children are concerned? There is absolutely no doubt in any clear thinking individual's mind that heavy cigarette smoking is dangerous. It has been well over ten years since the Surgeon General's office released the report demonstrating the relationship between cigarette smoking and lung cancer, as well as its adverse effect on the cardiovascular system. Despite these proven threats to health, 3,200 new adolescents between the ages of twelve and eighteen take up smoking every single day. The strongest influence initiating this terrible habit has been shown to be smoking behavior of the parents.

The Academy of Pediatrics recently sent out a poster to all its members. This sign reads: "For the health of your children, please do not smoke."

What comes through loud and clear from all this is obvious—stop smoking cigarettes for your own sake as well as for the future health of your children.

Should I use bubble baths for my baby girl? I have been told that it can cause internal trouble.

Bubble baths are widely used. In the great majority of

cases they cause no harm. However, a small percentage of children do develop rashes from their use. These eruptions can appear on any part of the body that is exposed to the bubble bath material and are considered in the "contact dermatitis" group of skin rashes.

In my experience, the rash is the only side effect from the use of bubble bath. Very rarely girls do complain of burning and itching around the vagina. However, these symptoms do not represent any internal infection. When the bubble bath is discontinued, the rash and any symptoms associated with it promptly disappear. I am not aware of any case of vaginal or urinary tract infection related to the use of a bubble bath.

Should skim milk be used after discontinuing formula?

I do not recommend the use of skim milk upon discontinuing formula feeding. My routine is to switch from the formula (or breast milk) to regular whole milk. Not enough is known about the baby's specific nutritional requirements for me to advocate the complete elimination of fat at such a young age. As a colleague of mine recently said, "If God did not want babies to have some fat in their milk, breast milk would be fat-free," and, of course, breast milk does contain fat. Some nutritionists believe that skim milk may provide too much protein and salt and they prefer waiting until the baby is at least one year old before using it. I agree with this approach. The vitamin content of skim milk is not an issue—it has plenty of vitamins. The question is, rather, whether or not some fat in the milk is necessary for normal growth and development during the first year of life. If the baby is gaining weight too rapidly, I recommend diluting the regular whole milk in order to cut down on the calories. Other pediatricians use a 99 percent fat-free milk for the same purpose. I believe that by one year of age the obese baby can safely be given skim milk.

Occasionally, babies vomit up the whole milk, and in these cases the use of a modified skim milk product may be helpful. In a true milk allergy case, neither whole nor skim milk should be used. A milk substitute formula, such as one of the soybean preparations, should be given instead.

We are expecting our first baby, and I have just been informed that I have Rh-negative blood. What effects will this have on the baby and any other children we will have? Is there anything that can be done to safeguard our children before they are born?

If you have not had a previous miscarriage or abortion, you need not worry about the Rh factor with your first baby. If your husband is Rh-positive, there is a chance that subsequent babies will be affected. However, you will never have any problem as long as you receive an injection of Rhogam within forty-eight hours of delivery of this baby and after any other future babies.

The combination of an Rh-negative mother and an Rh-positive father may lead to trouble. This can cause a condition called *erythroblastosis fetalis*, in which the baby may be born jaundiced or may become jaundiced very shortly after birth because the red blood cells break down. If not treated properly, it can lead to brain damage. The idea is to prevent the jaundice from becoming too severe. The usual methods of treatment include the use of phototherapy lamps and exchange transfusions, both of which are quite effective.

Recently a revolutionary new method for preventing this problem from ever developing has been discovered and is currently being used widely. This is the use of Rhogam. The initial sensitization of Rh-negative mothers is prevented by the injection of this specific gamma globulin. All Rh-negative mothers should be given an injection of this material shortly after delivering their first babies and after each subsequent delivery. By so doing, none of the babies will develop jaundice due to Rh incompatibility. The sensitization process is not allowed to take place. Rhogam cannot help the Rh-negative woman who has already had children, since she has already been sensitized.

My 2 1/2-year-old daughter has been masturbating since she was two months old. My doctor told me to just ignore her and not spank her for it. I would appreciate any opinion or information you could give.

Your doctor is absolutely right. The best approach to masturbation is to ignore it. This is a harmless habit and does not hurt the baby in any way. You should never scold, spank, or threaten the child. It is terribly wrong to make your baby feel guilty about this habit. In my experience, infants and small children always stop masturbating, sooner or later.

Masturbation is not that uncommon and occurs in female infants much more often than in males. It is important to remember that masturbation is not associated with any psychological or emotional problems. I remember a concerned mother telling me: "I am sure that my Suzy is oversexed. She masturbates so often." Well, Suzy was fifteen months old at the time and perfectly normal and healthy in every way. And, of course, there is no such thing as an oversexed fifteen-month-old.

My eighteen-month-old baby refuses to eat her solid food, except for a few spoonfuls. What should I do?

First of all, let me assure you that your child will not starve. This may sound silly and facetious, but you would be amazed to know that many mothers are really convinced that this can occur. It just never happens. When your child gets hungry enough she will eat. The sooner you stop forcing, yelling, screaming, punishing, etc., the sooner the problem will be resolved, and the better off both you and your child will be.

As far as your baby is concerned, let me now get a bit more specific. Cut down on the quantity of milk that you give her each day to a maximum of three glasses. It is a well-known fact that children who are overly dependent on milk for their caloric intake do not have much appetite for solid food. This may be the problem with your child. In addition, a child who only drinks milk and little else can develop an iron-deficiency anemia. The next thing to do is to completely eliminate the so-called junk foods—cookies, potato chips, pretzels, soda, etc. Present her with three well-balanced meals each day, and do not force her to eat any of it. I can guarantee that if she does not eat the junk foods between meals, she will get hungry enough to eat some of the nutritionally sound foods you prepare. There is no law that says she needs to clean her plate. Your child should not be made to feel guilty when she does not eat nor should she be praised or rewarded when she does eat. Relax and stop worrying so much. You will be pleasantly surprised with the change in your child's eating patterns and habits if you follow the simple advice I have given.

I have been reading about the beneficial effects of taking very large doses of vitamins. Do you think that we should give our baby extra vitamins in order to build up her resistance to infection?

No, you should not. It certainly is true that much has been written recently about the use of megavitamins and all the miraculous results that follow. Massive doses of vitamin C are supposed to prevent colds. Huge doses of multi-vitamins have been reported effective in treating childhood psychosis and learning disabilities. As far as I am concerned, this is all unproven. There is absolutely no scientific proof that these tremendous doses of vitamins do any good at all. In fact, there is evidence that this form of "therapy" may indeed be harmful. I would especially be careful about giving your baby extra-large doses of vitamins A and D. Overdoses of these two vitamins can be quite dangerous. My best advice is to simply give the baby her regular daily dose of multi-vitamin drops and leave it at that.

I take my two-year-old to a day-care center that has a large number of children. Since he is exposed to so many other youngsters, aren't his chances of getting an infection greater than if he were put in a family-type day-care house with fewer children?

Until very recently, I would have agreed that this would be the case. But a recent interesting study conducted in Sweden has changed my thinking. My answer now is that your child is probably not more susceptible to infection in the larger day-care center. Swedish physicians studied this question by following three separate groups of children. The first group went to day-care centers that had between sixteen and sixty-eight children. The second group evaluated went to family day-care centers that each had a total of four children. The third group of children studied stayed in their own homes. The results were as follows: As might be expected, the children remaining at home had the least number of respiratory infections. But interestingly enough, the other two groups (day-care centers and family centers) had the same number of infections. I would, therefore, not worry about the actual number of children in the day-care center that you use, but I would rather concern myself with the quality of the personnel taking care of your child.

I am worried about my baby's tongue. It has a number of raised patches on it and looks a bit like a map. What could this be?

You are probably describing what we call a "geographic" tongue. This type of tongue has a number of smooth patches that are easily seen on top. These areas may be bright red with yellowish or whitish margins, and the rest of the tongue has the usual roughened appearance. Since these patches are often confluent (maplike), the name commonly used is a geographic tongue. It does not bother the baby in the least. The cause is unknown and there is absolutely no treatment for it. It may last for many months, but eventually it disappears.

My one-month-old baby girl has a bunch of tiny whitish dots on her forehead and nose. I am very worried about this rash. What should I do about it?

Stop worrying. It sounds to me as if your baby has miliaria, a harmless rash caused by an obstruction of the sweat glands. The chances are that if you simply cool off the room and keep less clothes and blankets on her, the rash will fade away. Miliaria appears over the face when a baby is kept too warm and perspires. It does not hurt the baby in any way, and no treatment other than cooling off the baby is necessary.

While we are on the subject of overheated babies, the other common rash that often develops from this is prickly heat. This rash usually appears over the head, neck, and shoulders and is made up of bunches of small red dots. Again, there is no reason to worry. Cool off your baby and presto—the rash magically disappears.

My two-week-old boy holds his head tilted to one side all the time. Why is he doing this, and what can I do about it?

I would suggest that you have your baby's doctor check it out. It sounds as if your young man has a wry neck, or what technically is called "torticollis." This condition is not uncommon and in most cases clears up without any specific treatment. The usual cause is an overpull on a muscle on one side of the infant's neck during delivery. This can result in some damage and shortening of that neck muscle ("sternocleidomastoid"), and often a distinct lump can be felt in the muscle. If this is the case, simple muscle-stretching exercises help clear it up. This is carried out by your pushing the baby's head in the opposite lateral direction fifteen or twenty times, two or three times a day. If, for example, your baby's head is tilted to the right, firmly push it to the left. The baby may object, since his position of comfort is to the right side. The lump in the muscle disappears within a month or two. But to be completely on the safe side, have your doctor examine the baby. Severe cases of torticollis may require surgical correction.

Can a newborn baby hear?

Yes, he can. Actual testing within the first month of life is not easy, but it can be done by a skilled otolaryngologist (ear, nose, and throat specialist) with proper equipment. If there is any question at all in your mind about your baby's hearing, it is very important that this be discussed with your doctor. Observant parents often notice a hearing problem before the baby's doctor discovers it. There are certain situations in which hearing problems are more common. Premature babies, babies born to mothers having German measles early during the pregnancy, and babies coming from families with congenital hearing problems must be watched extra carefully. Danger signals that might point to hearing difficulties include:

1) A newborn baby who does not startle in response to a sharp clap within three to six feet of him

2) A two-month-old who does not waken from a sudden loud noise in his room

3) A four-month-old who does not turn to the source of a distinct sound

4) A six-month-old who gradually stops his babbling noises

5) An eight-month-old who does not enjoy ringing a bell or shaking a rattle

6) A twelve-month-old who does not start imitating the sounds that his parents make to him

It is very important that an early diagnosis of a hearing

difficulty be made. For best results, hearing aids must be applied as early as possible. We recently had such a case, and a hearing aid was started at six months of age. The little fellow is doing fine.

I am due to give birth next month. If it is a boy, do you suggest that he be circumcised?

If you had asked me that question two years ago the answer would have been easy and it would have been yes, but as of today the answer is more complicated. The Academy of Pediatrics has recently officially stated that there is no absolute medical indication for routine circumcision in the newborn. On the other hand, the American Academy of Obstetrics and Gynecology has thus far declined to endorse this statement. So where do we stand? Everybody would agree about a circumcision for religious reasons. Aside from the religious or ritual circumcision, the decision as to whether or not a newborn boy should be circumcised now remains with the parents. There are pros and cons and two distinct schools of thought. On the one hand, the uncircumcised boy requires more careful attention to personal hygiene of the penis in order to prevent infection. Another factor is the possible concern of the uncircumcised boy who does not look like his circumcised father. Weighed against this are the possible complications of the procedure itself, namely, local infection to the area or bleeding.

When I was in medical school, we were taught that noncircumcision might lead to cancer of the prostate or to cancer of the cervix for the mates of the uncircumcised males. We also learned that circumcision protects against cancer of the penis. However, current medical evidence refutes all this and points to the fact that there are no real *medical* indications for circumcision. All would agree that circumcision in the delivery room right after birth is wrong and should never be done. If a newborn is to be circumcised, he should be at least twenty-four hours old at the time it is performed.

A final word about this subject. My own personal experience would lead me to suggest circumcision if the final decision were left up to me. I personally have not seen any complications from the procedure. On the other hand, I have seen many uncircumcised young adults during my stint in the U. S. Navy who developed severe infections around the foreskin, and these infections required circumcision. There is no question that the adult circumcision is a more difficult and painful procedure than that of the newborn.

My baby hiccups all the time. Is there anything wrong with her? What can I do about it?

During the first few months of life, many babies do a great deal of hiccuping, especially after feedings. This is absolutely normal, and no treatment is indicated. Hiccups do not bother the infant in any way. My best advice is to ignore the whole thing. After the first few months, the hiccuping becomes less and less frequent.

My newborn boy has very swollen breasts. What is the matter with him?

Nothing is the matter with him. Many newborns, both boys and girls, develop swollen breasts shortly after birth. In some cases a watery, milky fluid is excreted from the nipples of the swollen breasts. This is all perfectly normal and does not mean that your baby is sick. The swelling is caused by a small amount of the mother's female hormones passing into the baby's bloodstream at birth. Leave the breasts alone. Never squeeze or massage them—this can cause an infection. It all clears up in a very short period of time.

My two-month-old baby boy does an awful lot of sneezing. Does this mean he has a cold?

Sneezing by itself, no matter how frequent, does not mean that your baby has a cold. I would say that during the first three or four months of their lives the majority of babies sneeze very frequently, and this can be considered normal. The sneezing is usually caused by either dust or some dried mucus in the nose. This tickles the baby and triggers a sneeze. A good, vigorous sneeze will often efficiently blow out the mucus or dust. If your baby does not have a running nose or fever and is taking his feedings without difficulty, the chances are he does not have a cold. In other words, sneezing that is not associated with other signs and symptoms of illness is no cause for concern.

At what age will I be able to tell for sure the color of my new baby's eyes?

Most babies are born with slate-colored eyes (sort of a gray-blue color). Gradually, pigment is deposited in the iris. By the time the baby is about one year of age, his eyes have turned to their permanent color.

I heard that it is unhealthy to cut my baby's nails. What do you think about this?

I think that whoever told you that doesn't know what he is talking about. It is important to cut your baby's nails, both finger- and toenails, just as soon and just as often as they need cutting. If you allow the nails to grow too long before cutting them, the baby can easily scratch himself. I remember one little baby who actually injured the inside of his eye with his own sharp fingernail. I would suggest that a two-person approach be used when it comes to cutting your baby's nails—one holder and one cutter. Nail clippers or cuticle scissors may be used. Actually, the best time to do the job is when the baby is asleep.

My baby has an umbilical hernia. Her grandmother advises that I use a belly band. What do you think?

Tell grandma that belly bands (as well as coins, adhesive tape, etc.) should never be used. All they do is hide the hernia, and the skin underneath may become irritated and infected. It has definitely been proven that all these methods do not help close the hernia. In practically all cases, umbilical hernias, whatever their size, close up by themselves by the time the baby is two years old. This type of hernia never causes the baby any discomfort or trouble. Contrary to what you may have heard, crying does not aggravate the condition. It is true that while the baby is crying, the hernia may push out a bit further, but this makes no difference as far as when the hernia finally will disappear. It is of interest that umbilical hernias are more common in black babies than in white babies. Occasionally, a black baby will require a simple surgical procedure to close the hernia if it has not closed off by two years of age. Surgical corrections of umbilical hernias in white babies are very rare indeed. In any case, if the umbilical hernia has not reduced itself by the time your baby is two years old, a surgeon should be consulted.

My baby's chin quivers, and his hands and feet shake. Does this mean he is nervous and high-strung?

No, it does not. These trembling movements are common during the first few months. Your baby's nervous system is not completely developed, and so he has these exaggerated responses to various stimuli. This kind of trembling usually happens when the baby is excited or startled by a sudden noise or when he is suddenly cooled. These trembling movements are normal, and nothing need be done about them except to stop worrying. As the baby gets older, his nervous system matures, and the quivering and trembling stops.

I just brought my new baby girl home from the hospital. She has a bloody vaginal discharge. Is this normal?

Yes, it is. A fair number of newborn girls do have a vaginal discharge during the first week or two. This discharge may be bloody or it may be whitish. It may be profuse or it may be scanty. No matter what, it is no cause for alarm. The vaginal discharge is due to a hormonal effect from the mother. The discharge stops by itself without any treatment, and it does not recur.

I have been told that talcum powder can be dangerous for my baby—that it can cause pneumonia and even cancer. Is this true?

No, it is not. Talc properly used is absolutely harmless. I have reviewed the literature on this subject and have found that there is no evidence at all to support the belief that the use of talcum powder can hurt the baby. As a matter of fact, epidemiologic studies involving modern talc miners who spend their lives mining this material have not shown an increased incidence of cancer. Obviously, if an entire can of talcum powder is accidentally poured down a baby's throat, it will cause the baby to choke. But if talc is applied in the normal manner, it is safe.

One of my baby's eyes waters and tears all the time, and sometimes whitish material collects in the inner corner of that eye. Why is this happening, and what can I do about it?

Your baby has a blocked tear duct. This is quite common and almost always clears up by itself before the baby is one year old. Normally, tears travel from the eye through the open tear duct into the nasal cavity. When this duct is partially or completely plugged up, the tears cannot drain off into the nose and so fill up in the eye and overflow and run down the cheek. Due to the blocked drainage, an irritation and infection can develop. Thick white or yellow or green material may accumulate in the inner corner of the eye. If this happens, your doctor should be called so that he may prescribe appropriate eye drops.

In the great majority of cases, the blocked tear duct opens by itself and requires no specific treatment. If the duct is still plugged by the time your baby is one year old, an eye doctor should be consulted. He may have to surgically probe open the duct, and this would require a brief stay in the hospital. This procedure is safe and easy. I would suggest that when whitish material accumulates in the inner corner of the eye, it be wiped away with a moist cotton ball from the outer corner of the eye inward toward the nose and then down the side of the nose. This method sometimes helps to open the plugged tear duct.

How should I clean my baby's ears?
Very carefully. In my experience, the overvigorous use of cotton swabs can damage the ear canal and even the eardrum. I have seen a number of babies brought to the office actually bleeding from the ear canal after a cleaning. I don't remember where I heard the following advice but I agree with it: "The *smallest* object you should ever put into your baby's ear is your elbow." I suggest that you use a moistened cotton swab and gently clean around the opening of the ear canal. Don't ever poke the swab deep into the canal. Don't worry about the accumulation of earwax—it will either come out by itself or will dissolve. Rarely, it may be necessary for your physician to actually remove the wax. Leave that job to the doctor.

My newborn baby has a large lump on his head that my doctor called a cephalohematoma. What is it and is it dangerous?
A cephalohematoma is a localized accumulation of blood and fluid under the scalp that is formed by pressure at the time of the delivery. A cephalohematoma is not at all dangerous. This swelling may remain for weeks or even months but always clears up. It does not bother the baby and does not cause brain damage or any other problem. No treatment is indicated. Just leave it alone, and it will gradually be absorbed and disappear.

What is the soft spot on top of my baby's head, and when does it close up?
The soft spot (called the *anterior fontanel*) is the area on top of the baby's head where the skull bones have not yet completely come together. The anterior fontanel gradually becomes smaller and usually is completely closed some time between twelve to eighteen months of age. Let me add that you cannot hurt your baby by

combing or cleaning over this soft spot. Many new parents are unnecessarily worried about this.

What is cradle cap, and what can I do about it?

Cradle cap is a condition in which yellowish, greasy crusts form on the baby's scalp. Most of the time it develops because the scalp is not cleaned properly. It frequently forms over the soft spot ("anterior fontanel") because parents are afraid to rub too hard over that area. Occasionally, cradle cap may be caused by a form of eczema called seborrheic eczema. In such cases, scaling may also be found behind the baby's ears. If this happens, your doctor may wish to prescribe a specific ointment to help clear it up. Simple cradle cap is easily gotten rid of by rubbing oil into the area, then using a fine-tooth comb to loosen the crusts followed by shampooing the head. One or two such treatments usually do the trick.

My one-week-old has a pinkish, round piece of tissue protruding up from her umbilical cord area. What is this, and what should I do about it?

It sounds to me as if your baby has an umbilical granuloma. It looks like a little pink mushroom on a thin stalk. There is no reason to panic. Granulomas are seen fairly often and are easily treated. Simply keep the area clean with alcohol. These extra pieces of tissue usually dry up and fade away in a few days. Some granulomas persist and become moist and inflamed. In such cases your doctor may want to cauterize the granuloma with a silver nitrate stick. This is a simple office procedure and is quite effective. Rarely, the granuloma is too large to be cauterized, and your doctor will tie it off at its base. It will then fall off.

Is air conditioning harmful for my new baby?

Absolutely not. If the weather is such that you would be more comfortable in an air-conditioned room, the same holds true for your new baby. Please remember that your baby's temperature is no different from yours. As a matter of fact, most hospital nurseries nowadays are air-conditioned, so that it is foolish for you to believe that it would be harmful for your infant. A baby is much more comfortable and content in a cool environment, rather than in a hot, stuffy room.

I have been told that my baby has thrush. What causes thrush, and what can I do about it?

Thrush is an infection of the mouth caused by monilia—a yeastlike organism. It is fairly common during the first weeks of life. Whitish patches are seen on the baby's tongue and inside the cheeks and lips. If you cannot easily scrape this white material off, it is probably thrush and not milk curd. Your doctor should be notified so that he may prescribe the appropriate medication to get rid of it. Treatment is effective, and the thrush can be eliminated in a very few days.

Thrush is picked up by the infant during delivery as he or she passes through the mother's vagina. It usually does not show up until the baby is home from the hospital.

I think that my seven-month-old's eyes look crossed. Is this anything to worry about?

In many cases, a baby's eyes may look crossed but actually are not. The optical illusion of crossed eyes is created by the fold of skin extending from the bridge of the baby's nose across the inner corner of the eye (these are called *epicanthic folds*) that is prominent in many infants.

Your doctor should be able to differentiate true crossed eyes, or "squint," from the prominent epicanthic fold situation. A true squint must be treated by an ophthalmologist just as soon as the diagnosis is made, no matter how young the baby may be at the time. Early treatment is very important in order to prevent loss of vision in the crossed eye. The crossed eye is not being used to see, and if this is allowed to go on for too long, loss of vision in that eye can result.

During the first few months of life, it is common for a baby's eyes to turn once in awhile, and this may be considered normal. If, on the other hand, they turn in or out all or most of the time, your doctor should be told about it. This holds true no matter what the age of the infant. Often a baby's eyes will cross only when he is looking at an object that he is holding. This is okay. His arm is just too short as he tries to focus on the object held too close to him.

My seven-month-old wants to stand. Will this cause him to be bowlegged?

No, it will not. If he wants to stand, let him do so. The more exercise the better. If he is happy standing, so be it. Despite what Grandma may tell you to the contrary, standing will not lead to bowlegs.

Many babies have a normal amount of bowing of their legs which gradually disappears. I have never seen a case of bowlegs due to vitamin deficiency (rickets). Another point to remember is that bowlegs often run in families. Just remember that there is no relationship between bowing and standing.

When can we travel with our new baby?

Anytime you feel like it. There is no medical reason that prevents you from taking a new baby on a trip by car, plane, or train. Just as long as you make proper preparations for feedings, diaper changes, etc., your new baby can travel at any age. As a matter of fact, little babies are usually very good travelers.

My doctor just told me that my baby has a functional heart murmur and that there is nothing to worry about. I am frightened out of my mind about this. Please tell me if there really is no reason for me to be concerned.

Your doctor is 100 percent correct. A functional murmur does not mean a thing, and you can relax and forget about it. In my experience, there is nothing more frightening to parents than to be told that their baby has a heart murmur. In the great majority of cases, these murmurs are indeed functional and absolutely harmless. But the word "heart murmur" strikes terror in the hearts of parents, and it is very difficult to convince these mothers and fathers that there really is nothing for them to worry about.

There are two separate and distinct types of heart murmur: (1) functional (a better word being "innocent") and (2) organic. The functional or innocent murmur is normal, whereas the organic heart murmur represents some disease of the heart. Therefore, what is most important is for your doctor to determine whether your baby's murmur is innocent or organic. He can do this by a careful physical examination, with certain laboratory tests such as an electrocardiogram if he feels they are necessary. If he then tells you that your baby has a functional or innocent murmur, that should be the end of it. About one in three children has this type of murmur. In some studies the incidence of the innocent murmur is as high as 50 percent. On the other hand, only about six out of one thousand babies have an organic heart murmur.

What is most disturbing to me is the large number of children with innocent murmurs who lead unnecessarily restricted lives. This may be due to misdiagnosis, in which an innocent murmur is called an organic murmur, but usually the problem is caused by the parents. Even though the doctor reassures them that there is nothing to worry about, they just don't believe that a "murmur" can be normal. They then take it upon themselves to restrict the child's activities, and this causes all sorts of unnecessary psychological and emotional problems. This misunderstanding on the part of the family may be due to inconclusive medical advice given to them. The doctor must take enough time, not only to tell the parents that the murmur is functional, but to be absolutely sure that they understand that this type of murmur does not mean that there is anything wrong with the baby's heart. In many cases these innocent murmurs disappear as the child gets older, but it really makes no difference whether or not they do.

We still do not know what actually causes the innocent murmur. There are many theories, but the exact mechanism is unclear. What is certain, however, is that the child's heart is completely normal. No special supervision is necessary, and there should be no restriction of activity for the child with an innocent or functional murmur.

Can we use flashbulbs to take pictures of our new baby?

Yes, you certainly can. There is no danger of injuring your baby's eyes; so go right ahead and click away. I hope your pictures come out sharp and clear.

My newborn baby does not have any tears when she cries. Is this normal?

Yes, this is perfectly normal. Most newborns do not have tears immediately after birth. It usually takes a few months before you actually will see tears trickle down your baby's face when she cries.

When should our baby start wearing shoes?

Your baby should get his first pair of shoes when he has started to take a few steps by himself. In my experience, most parents are in too great a hurry. As soon as the baby starts pulling himself up to a standing position, they assume that the baby needs shoes. This is just not so. There is no rush. It's healthier for your baby's feet if you wait. Until your baby actually walks by himself, let him stay barefoot or with some type of booty to cover his feet when outdoors. The baby who stands barefoot or walks around holding on to the furniture without shoes is getting good exercise for his foot arch muscles. Most orthopedists believe that it is healthier for a baby to remain barefoot until he is actually walking by himself, and I agree.

When it is time to get the first pair of shoes, the important thing is to make sure that they fit properly. This first walker should have a semisoft sole so that the baby's feet still get a good amount of exercise while walking. Even when the baby already has shoes, you should continue to let him walk around barefoot in the house part of each day.

My baby has a small split in the skin around his anus. What is this, and how serious is it?

You are describing what is called an anal fissure (or fissure *in ano*). We see this fairly often in infants and small children, and it is not serious. It usually is caused by the baby's straining while having a bowel movement or by the overzealous cleaning of the anal area. Sometimes there is no explanation for the fissure. Bright red blood is seen on the surface of the stool, or you may find some red blood on the tissue or on whatever else you use to clean the baby's bottom after a stool. A careful examination of the anal area will demonstrate a small crack in the skin. Treatment of the anal fissure consists of frequently applying a simple healing ointment to the involved area and sitting the baby in a warm bath two or three times a day. In most cases this will quickly heal the fissure.

My three-year-old has had his elbow dislocated three separate times. Each time my doctor simply snapped it back into place. I actually heard a click when the doctor turned his arm. Can I do anything to prevent this from happening again?

You are describing a condition called subluxation of the head of the radius. This most often happens to children between two and five years of age and is hardly ever seen after the child is eight years old. The usual story is that the child has had his hand and arm forcibly jerked by a taller person. Most of the time this occurs when an adult and child are walking along the street, and, for one reason or another, the child's hand is suddenly yanked (for example, at street corners to stop the child from walking out into traffic). The youngster immediately starts to cry, and his arm hangs limply at his side, slightly flexed at the elbow. He tries very hard not to move the arm in any direction, since this causes him great pain. With subluxation of the radius, X rays are not necessary. A simple maneuver to reduce the dislocation at the elbow can be performed by the doctor in his office. As soon as the arm is snapped back into place, the child has no further pain and can move his arm around as good as new. This condition is often recurrent. The only advice I can give you to help prevent it from happening again is to be especially careful not to jerk or yank your child's arm. In any event, it will not be a problem when your child gets older. Subluxation of the radius does not weaken or damage the affected arm.

What are my chances of having twins?

The actual incidence of twins in the United States is reported as one in eighty-six births. Of these, about 75 percent are fraternal ("polyovular") and 25 percent are identical ("monovular"). The incidence of triplets is one in 7,000, and the incidence of quadruplets is one in 625,000.

In the case of identical twins—twins that come from the same egg—there are no known causes; it just happens. As far as fraternal twins are concerned, we do know that a family history of twins increases your chances. Another important factor that might lead to fraternal twins, or even triplets, is the use of fertility drugs. Women who have had trouble conceiving and are placed on a fertility drug have a higher incidence of multiple births than the general population. We also find fraternal twins more often after the second pregnancy and in older women.

Identical twins are always of the same sex and grow up the same size and often with the same temperament. They really are identical in that strangers have a hard time telling them apart. As a matter of fact, I recently had a set of identical twins whom the father could not tell apart for many months.

Fraternal twins may or may not be of the same sex. There is no problem in telling them apart. By examining the placenta after delivery, your doctor can usually determine whether or not you have identical or fraternal twins. There are cases, however, in which the doctor may not be sure. In these cases, by two to four years of age you will be able to see that the fraternal twins have important physical differences.

How can I tell if my newborn will be right- or left-handed?

There is no way to determine the handedness of your baby for the first year or two. Most small babies are ambidexterous until around four years of age. You may get a clue by carefully observing your baby's hands to see if he uses one of them more often than the other to hold, point, or reach.

Handedness is primarily an heredity trait, and environment is only a secondary factor. There is a specific center of the brain for handedness, and this center is genetically determined. My own family is a good example of the genetics of handedness. My father was left-handed, my mother right-handed, and both my brother and I are left-handed. My wife and I are both left-handed, and one of our two children is left-handed. This adds up to five out of seven left-handed Edens. Compare this to the general population, where only 6 to 8 percent is left-handed, and you can see that handedness runs in families.

Some people believe that we live in a right-handed world, but I obviously do not agree. As a matter of fact, sometimes left-handedness can be an advantage, as, for example, in playing tennis. I am at a distinct advantage, since most of my tennis opponents are not accustomed to playing left-handed people; besides, being left-handed has not hurt Jimmy Connors or Rod Laver one bit.

But, more important, it is unhealthy to try to change a child who is naturally left-handed. This really can cause problems, including stuttering (from the tension the change places the child under), mirror writing, writer's cramp, and more. Whatever hand your child uses, so be it. This has been genetically determined, and you have no business interfering with the natural course of events.

Is it true that the "hyperactive" child can be helped with a special diet?

This is a hard question to answer. All the returns are as yet not in. There is no question that the hyperactive or hyperkinetic child is difficult to treat. There has been a lot of recent publicity, including a number of books, claiming dramatic improvement in symptoms with the use of special diets. Many parents with hyperactive children are anxious to use these special diets. The Committee on Nutrition of the American Academy of Pediatrics has recently reported that so far there is "no evidence that dietary modification plays a role in the treatment of children with hyperkinesis." The committee also states that further investigations must be conducted before firm conclusions can be reached. I agree with their position. I would like to see more controlled studies proving that these diets are effective before I recommend that they be used.

What is crib death?

Crib death refers to the sudden unexpected death of an infant between one and five months of age, almost always during sleep, which is unexplained by history and in which a thorough autopsy fails to demonstrate any cause for the death. Another name for crib death is "sudden infant death syndrome." The usual story is that an infant is put to bed perfectly well, and the following morning he is found dead in his crib.

The incidence of crib death is about two out of one

thousand babies. There are many possible theories to explain it, but thus far no definite cause has been implicated. It may well be that there are a number of different causes. A tremendous amount of research is being done in this area to try to find the cause and, more important, to try to find ways to prevent it from happening. However, as of now there is no way for parents or doctors to prevent crib death.

Is there anything I can do to prevent my baby from developing hardening of the arteries and heart disease when he grows up?

I think you can. There are a number of proven risk factors that predispose the adult to developing hardening of the arteries and subsequent heart disease. Theoretically, preventing these risk factors in children may help to slow down the atherosclerotic process. I should like to emphasize that the effectiveness of this has not been proven, but it makes good sense to me to try prevention anyway. The factors that may make the child susceptible to later atherosclerosis (and which you can do something about) are:

1) Obesity: The fat child is more likely to become the fat adult, and so it is important not to allow your infant to gain weight too rapidly.

2) High salt intake: This may predispose your child to the later development of high blood pressure, which can lead to heart disease.

3) Exercise: It has been shown that sedentary people have a greater chance of suffering heart attacks than those who exercise regularly. It is, therefore, important to encourage your small child to exercise so that this will become a way of life for him.

There is one additional factor that may be significant, and that is smoking by the mother during her pregnancy. Some evidence has accumulated suggesting that this may damage the developing arterial circulation of the fetus. This can be the first step toward the development of later atherosclerosis. Again, this has not been proven, but my own feeling is why take a chance?

Can drugs that I take during my pregnancy harm my newborn?

Yes, certain drugs can damage the developing fetus. This does not happen very often, but the possibility does exist. A number of drugs have been found to cause prenatal injury ("teratogenic"). The most dramatic example of such a drug is thalidomide. You probably remember the recent tragic situation in Europe when a large number of babies were born with absent limbs (called *amelia*) or with other limb defects. It was definitely proven that this occurred after the pregnant women had taken thalidomide during the first weeks of their pregnancies. We were very fortunate here in the United States that this drug was not yet commercially available. The Food and Drug Administration wanted further testing before allowing it to be distributed, and we should all be very grateful for their caution.

Other drugs that may on occasion damage the fetus are dicumarol, estrogens, androgens, and iodides. Since it is difficult to be sure that *any* drug is not potentially harmful to an embryo, I would strongly advise you to restrict any drug intake during your pregnancy, and only take those medications that are clearly necessary for your health. Always check with your physician before taking any drug while you are pregnant. This is by far the safest approach.

The lips of my baby girl's vagina are stuck together. What should I do about it?

You are describing "vulvar fusion." This is a condition in which there may be complete or incomplete fusion of the baby's vaginal lips. Even when this fusion is complete, there never is a problem as far as the baby's being able to urinate. Leave it alone. It almost always opens by itself later on in childhood. Some doctors advocate the use of hormonal creams to help open the fused area. In my experience, these creams are not necessary.

EPILOGUE

All of us have a great feeling of security when we know what to expect ahead of time. Surprises are fine at birthday parties but are not so fine when they involve new babies. The purpose of the *Handbook for New Parents* is to eliminate doubts and worries about your newborn. If you have read it through, you should be better prepared for the job at hand.

Twenty-five years of pediatric experience have been distilled into this book. I believe that all the important questions have been included.

It is essential that you give your baby the best possible start. There is no question in my mind that good parenting begins with being able to relax and actually enjoy your new baby. I hope this book will help you do just that.

INDEX

Abdominal distention, 26
ABO incompatability, 170-71
Accidents, 26-27
  prevention, 82-89
Air conditioning, 58, 192-93
Allergy, 155
  milk, 121, 179-80
American Academy of
  Pediatrics, 16, 32, 178
  Committee on Nutrition,
    47, 50-51, 200
American Board of
  Pediatrics, 16
Ammonia rash, 111
Anal fissure, 197
Anemia, iron deficiency,
  50-51, 161-62
Anterior fontanel, 24, 191-92
Antibiotics, 132
Antibodies, 30
  antipyretics, 145, 151
Appetite, 24-25, 47, 50-51
Automobile safety
  precautions, 87-88

Baby food, 49
Baby's room, 57-58
Bathing, 39, 178-79
Bile, 121, 126
Bilirubin, 167-68, 171-72
Birthmarks, 176
Blankets, 62

Bottle, 43, 44, 45, 46, 47, 72
Bowel movements, 41, 62, 78,
  124-28, 129-30
Breast-feeding, 43-45, 47, 48,
  72, 172
Breasts, infant's swollen, 187
Breath holding, 159-62
Breathing, 23-24
Bubble baths, 178-79
Burns, 27, 25-26

Cephalohematoma, 191
Cheesing, 119, 120
Chin quivering, 189
Cigarettes, 177-78, 201-02
Circumcision, 186-87
Clothing, 62
Colds, 79, 153-58, 183, 187-88
Colic, 61, 114-17
Conjugation, 168
Consciousness, loss of, 27
Constipation, 19, 25-26,
  124-28
Convulsions, 26, 159
  fever, 147-52
Coughs, 24, 78-79, 154, 157
Cradle cap, 42, 192
Cretinism, 21
Crib death, 200-01
Crying, 24, 41, 45-46, 58, 159
  causes, 59-63

207

INDEX

Cup, 50
Cuts, 26, 86–87

Day care centers, 183
Dehydration, 134–36
Diaper, 45, 61–62
    rash, 42, 109–13
Diarrhea, 25, 129–36
    causes, 131–32
Diptheria, 30, 33
Doctor
    giving information to, 27–38
    monthly visits, 18–22
    selecting, 11–17
    when to call, 23–28
    See also Pediatrician
D.P.T. shots, 33
    reaction, 34
Drowsiness, unusual, 25
Drugs and pregnancy, 202

Ears, 42
    cleaning, 191
Elbow dislocation, 197–98
Emergencies, 27
Encephalitis, 33
Epicanthic fold, 193
Epilepsy, 147–48
Erythroblastosis, fetalis, 180–81
Exchange transfusion, 170
Exercise, 201
Eyes, 38, 42
    color, 188
    crossed, 193–94
    mucus, 42
    tears, 63, 196
    vision, 38
    watering, 190–91

Family physician, 13
Father, 96–100
Fatigue, 60
Feeding, 39–40, 43–52, 56, 119, 120
    amount, 46–47
    length, 71
    schedule, 45–46
Fennel seed tea, 116
Fever, 26, 27, 79–80, 142–46, 154, 156
    convulsions, 147
    as immunization reaction, 34
    vs. temperature, 137
First month, 37–42
Flashbulbs, 196
Foman, Dr. S. J., 47
Formula, 47, 51, 179–80

Gastrointestinal infections, 132
German measles, 30, 33

Handedness, 199–200
Head
    injuries, 163–66
    lump on, 191
    soft spot, 24, 191–92
    tilted, 184–85
Hearing, 38, 185–86
Heart disease prevention, 201–02
Heart murmur
    functional, 194–96
    organic, 195
Hemangiomas, 176
Hernia, 63
    inguinal, 176–77
    umbilical, 188–89
Hiccuping, 24, 41, 187

INDEX

Hippocrates, 130
Hunger, 60
Hydrocele, 176
Hydrocephalus, 20
Hyperactivity, 200
Hypertonic infants, 61

Illness, 27, 62
Immunizations, 29-34
    reactions, 34
    schedule, 32-33
Injuries, 26-27
    head, 160-66
Ipecac, syrup of, 84-85
Iron supplements, 50-51
Irritability, 24, 61

Jaundice, 167-72, 180

Kernicterus, 169-70

Loneliness, 60-61

Masturbation, 181
Mattress, 57
Measles, 30, 31, 33
Meconium, 131
Megavitamins, 182
Miliaria, 184
Milk, 47-48, 50-51, 181-82
    allergy, 121, 179-80
    breast, 172, 179
    skim, 179-80
M.M.R. shot, 32-33
    reaction, 34
Monilia, 193
Mother, working, 101-06
Mumps, 30, 33

Nails, 188
Nose, 42
    runny, 156-57
Nurse-midwife, 13

Obesity, 46, 201
Obstetrician, 13-14
Overfeeding, 46, 131
Overheating, 62, 184

Pacifiers, 64-69, 72, 116
Parenteral disease, 132
Pediatric Annals, 88
Pediatrician, 13-14
    prenatal visit, 14-15
    rapport, 20-21
    training and affiliations, 15-16
    See also Doctor
Pertussis, 30, 32
Phenobarbital, 151-52
Pillow, 57
Phototherapy, 170
Physician (see Doctor)
Poisoning, 27
    antidotes, 84-85
    prevention, 83-85
Polio, 29, 30, 33
Pregnancy, 14, 33
    drugs and, 202
    smoking and, 177-78, 201-02
Prickly heat, 185

Rashes, 25, 42, 49, 79, 179
    white, 184
Rh incompatibility, 171, 180-81
Rhogam, 180
Rubella, 30, 33

INDEX

Salt, 47, 49, 201
Scalp, 42
Scrotum, 177
Shoes, 196-97
Skin, 23, 42
   color, 23
   mottling, 42
   jaundice, 167-72, 180
Sleep, 25, 53-58
   during first month, 40
Smallpox vaccination, 33
Smoking, 177-78, 201-02
Sneezing, 24, 41, 187-88
Solid foods, 48-49, 50, 51, 127, 133-34, 157, 181-82
   schedule, 48-49
Spitting up, 118-19, 120, 122-23
Spock, Dr., 106
Squint, 193-94
Standing, 194
Sternocleidomastoid, 184
Strawberry mark (see Hemangioma)
Subluxation, 197-98
Sugar, 49, 80, 127, 133
Sweat gland obstruction (see Miliaria)

Talcum powder, 190
Tear ducts, plugged, 190-91
Tears, 62-63, 196
Teeth, 46, 68, 74
   first, 175
Teething, 45, 76-81, 119, 131, 155
   remedy, 80
Temperature, 137-41. *See also* Fever
Testicles, 177

Tetanus, 30, 33, 87
Thalidomide, 202
Thermometer, 26, 138
Thrush, 193
Thumb sucking, 70-75
Toilet training, 90-95
Tongue
   geographic, 183-84
   tied, 175-76
   white patches on, 193
Torticollis, 184-85
Transfusion, exchange, 170
Travel, 194
Trembling, 189
Tuberculin test, 32, 34
Twins, 198-99

Umbilical cord, 39
Umbilical granuloma, 192
Upper respiratory infections (URI), 39, 183. *See also* Colds
Urination, 26, 41

Vaginal discharge, 189
Vitamins, 50, 182-83
Vomiting, 25, 118-23, 133, 154

Weaning, 48-49
Weight, 39, 52
Wheatley, Dr. George, 88
Whooping cough, 30, 33
Wilms' tumor, 19
World Health Organization, 32
Wry neck (see Torticollis)